200 NCLEX-Style Practice Questions: A Comprehensive Multi-Topic Nursing Review

Preparing for the NCLEX-RN® examination involves a comprehensive review of nursing fundamentals, medical-surgical topics, pharmacology, maternal-newborn care, pediatrics, mental health, leadership, and more. Beyond practicing with NCLEX-style questions, it's crucial to consult credible resources that align with current evidence-based guidelines and professional standards.

The **references** provided here offer a framework for in-depth study, covering everything from the official NCLEX test plan released by the National Council of State Boards of Nursing (NCSBN) to standard nursing textbooks and review guides. These resources reflect the key content areas tested on the NCLEX-RN and are frequently cited by nursing educators for their accuracy, depth, and alignment with the exam's structure.

As you prepare:

1. **Use the NCLEX Test Plan** to understand content weight and the types of questions you may encounter.
2. **Consult comprehensive review books** to practice test-taking strategies and question formats.

3. **Revisit core nursing textbooks** for detailed pathophysiology, interventions, and rationales.
4. **Refer to clinical guidelines** (CDC, AHA, ADA) for the most up-to-date best practices in infection control, emergency care, or chronic disease management.
5. **Check professional standards** from nursing organizations like ANA or AMSN to reinforce legal, ethical, and leadership concepts.

By integrating practice questions with these referenced materials, you can strengthen critical thinking skills, solidify foundational knowledge, and approach the NCLEX with confidence.

Disclaimer:

While these references reflect the general sources used in nursing education and NCLEX exam preparation, each practice question set is independently created for review purposes. Always consult your institution's guidelines, course textbooks, and the **latest** official NCLEX test plan for the most accurate and up-to-date information.

Q1.

A client is receiving intravenous heparin for the treatment of a deep vein thrombosis (DVT). Which laboratory test is most important to monitor for effectiveness of heparin therapy?

A. Prothrombin time (PT)
B. Platelet count
C. Activated partial thromboplastin time (aPTT)
D. International Normalized Ratio (INR)

Correct Answer: C. Activated partial thromboplastin time (aPTT)

Rationale:

- **Heparin** anticoagulation is monitored via the **aPTT**, which measures the intrinsic and common coagulation pathways.
- **PT** and **INR** monitor **warfarin** effectiveness.
- **Platelet count** is necessary to check for heparin-induced thrombocytopenia, but it doesn't measure the therapeutic level of heparin.

Q2.

A nurse is caring for a client with heart failure who takes furosemide daily. Which finding would require the **most immediate** nursing intervention?

A. Weight gain of 2 pounds in the last 24 hours
B. Potassium level of 3.2 mEq/L
C. Blood pressure of 138/88 mm Hg
D. Mild pedal edema at the end of the day

Correct Answer: B. Potassium level of 3.2 mEq/L

Rationale:

- **Hypokalemia** (< 3.5 mEq/L) is a significant adverse effect of **furosemide**, a loop diuretic. It can cause dangerous cardiac dysrhythmias and needs prompt intervention.
- A 2-pound weight gain in 24 hours is concerning for fluid retention in a heart failure client but not as immediately life-threatening as severe electrolyte imbalance.
- Mild pedal edema and a BP of 138/88 mm Hg are not as urgent compared to hypokalemia.

Q3.

A client with chronic obstructive pulmonary disease (COPD) reports increased dyspnea. The nurse notices the client is on 6 L/min nasal cannula of oxygen. Which intervention is **most appropriate**?

A. Increase oxygen flow rate to 10 L/min
B. Encourage pursed-lip breathing and reassess
C. Place the client in supine position
D. Decrease oxygen flow rate to 2 L/min

Correct Answer: B. Encourage pursed-lip breathing and reassess

Rationale:

- COPD clients benefit from **pursed-lip breathing** to promote better expiration and reduce air trapping.
- Increasing oxygen flow could diminish their respiratory drive if they retain CO_2.
- Supine positioning may worsen breathing.
- Decreasing oxygen to 2 L/min abruptly may cause hypoxia; the nurse should first use a noninvasive technique like pursed-lip breathing.

Q4.

A client with cirrhosis is receiving lactulose. Which finding indicates the medication is **effective**?

A. Decreased serum ammonia levels
B. Increased blood urea nitrogen (BUN)
C. Lower bilirubin levels
D. Increased urine output

Correct Answer: A. Decreased serum ammonia levels

Rationale:

- **Lactulose** is used to reduce **ammonia** levels in clients with liver dysfunction by promoting excretion via stools.
- BUN and bilirubin changes don't directly indicate lactulose effectiveness.
- While clients may have more bowel movements, it's the decrease in ammonia that shows true efficacy.

Q5.

A postoperative client has a sudden onset of chest pain and dyspnea. The nurse suspects a pulmonary embolism (PE). What is the **first** nursing action?

A. Call the healthcare provider immediately
B. Administer IV heparin
C. Elevate the head of the bed and apply supplemental oxygen
D. Check for a positive Homan's sign

Correct Answer: C. Elevate the head of the bed and apply supplemental oxygen

Rationale:

- In a suspected **PE**, the initial intervention is to **optimize oxygenation** and respiratory status—raise head of bed and give oxygen.
- The provider should be notified promptly, but the immediate nursing action is to address airway and breathing.
- IV heparin is commonly used for PE but only after obtaining provider orders.
- Homan's sign is unreliable and not a priority action.

Q6.

A client who has had a left-sided stroke presents with right-sided weakness. Which intervention is a **priority** to prevent joint contractures?

A. Keep the affected arm adducted and close to the body
B. Perform passive range-of-motion (ROM) exercises on the affected side
C. Place a pillow under the shoulder to elevate the joint
D. Limit use of the affected side to prevent overexertion

Correct Answer: B. Perform passive range-of-motion (ROM) exercises on the affected side

Rationale:

- After a stroke, **passive ROM exercises** help maintain joint mobility and prevent contractures.
- Keeping the arm constantly adducted or limiting use may worsen stiffness.
- Elevating the shoulder might help with edema but does not prevent

contractures as effectively as routine ROM.

Q7.

A client is admitted with acute pancreatitis. Which laboratory test would the nurse expect to be **most elevated**?

A. Serum lactate
B. Serum amylase
C. Serum calcium
D. Serum bilirubin

Correct Answer: B. Serum amylase

Rationale:

- **Amylase** and lipase levels are typically elevated in **acute pancreatitis**. Amylase is often significantly elevated in the early phase.
- Calcium may actually drop in pancreatitis.
- Bilirubin may rise if biliary obstruction is involved, but it's not the primary indicator.
- Lactate elevation could suggest poor tissue perfusion, not specifically pancreatitis.

Q8.

A client with chronic kidney disease (CKD) has a serum potassium of 6.2 mEq/L. Which intervention should the nurse anticipate?

A. Administer sodium polystyrene sulfonate (Kayexalate)
B. Restrict protein intake
C. Give oral potassium supplements
D. Increase IV fluids to 200 mL/hr

Correct Answer: A. Administer sodium polystyrene sulfonate (Kayexalate)

Rationale:

- **Kayexalate** helps remove **excess potassium** via the gastrointestinal tract in hyperkalemia.
- Restricting protein intake is a separate measure for CKD but doesn't acutely address hyperkalemia.
- Giving potassium supplements would worsen hyperkalemia.
- Increasing IV fluids alone won't sufficiently correct a dangerously high potassium.

Q9.

A client who underwent abdominal surgery two days ago has a sudden increase in wound drainage and the nurse sees bowel loops protruding from the incision site. What is the **priority** nursing action?

A. Apply a sterile saline dressing over the wound
B. Notify the surgeon
C. Raise the head of the bed to 90°
D. Gently reinsert the bowel and apply pressure

Correct Answer: A. Apply a sterile saline dressing over the wound

Rationale:

- Protrusion of bowel loops indicates **evisceration**, a surgical emergency. The **priority** is to cover the area with **sterile saline-soaked dressings** to prevent tissue drying and infection.
- The nurse should then call the provider.
- Do not attempt to reinsert the bowel.

Q10.

A postpartum client complains of **heavy lochia rubra** saturating one peri-pad every hour and passing several small clots. Her fundus is firm, midline, and located 1 cm below the umbilicus. Which action should the nurse take **first**?

A. Notify the healthcare provider
B. Massage the fundus vigorously
C. Assess the client's vital signs
D. Check the client's bladder for distension

Correct Answer: C. Assess the client's vital signs

Rationale:

- The fundus is firm, so uterine atony is less likely. Before calling the provider, the nurse should **assess vital signs** to evaluate hemodynamic stability.
- Other causes of postpartum hemorrhage (e.g., lacerations, retained fragments) might be considered, but the immediate nursing action is assessment of the mother's stability.

Q11.

A nurse is teaching a client about taking oral doxycycline for a respiratory infection. Which client statement indicates the need for **further teaching**?

A. "I should take this medication around the same time each day."
B. "I'll avoid direct sun and tanning beds while taking this medication."
C. "I can take this pill with a glass of milk to avoid an upset stomach."
D. "I should finish the entire prescription even if I feel better."

Correct Answer: C. "I can take this pill with a glass of milk to avoid an upset stomach."

Rationale:

- **Dairy products** can bind tetracyclines (like doxycycline) and reduce absorption.
- Taking it at consistent times daily helps maintain blood levels.
- Tetracyclines cause **photosensitivity**, so avoiding sun exposure is correct.
- Completing the full course is standard antibiotic teaching.

Q12.

A client with seizures is taking phenytoin. Which instruction should the nurse give about a potential side effect?

A. "You may experience excessive tearing from the eyes."
B. "Gum overgrowth can occur; regular dental care is essential."
C. "Light sensitivity is common; wear sunglasses indoors."
D. "Hair loss may occur but will return after treatment."

Correct Answer: B. "Gum overgrowth can occur; regular dental care is essential."

Rationale:

- **Phenytoin** is known for causing **gingival hyperplasia**. Good dental hygiene and regular dental check-ups are critical.
- Light sensitivity, excessive tearing, and hair loss are not classic phenytoin side effects.

Q13.

A client is prescribed metformin for type 2 diabetes. Which teaching point should the nurse emphasize?

A. "Take metformin on an empty stomach for best absorption."
B. "Stop taking metformin if you develop a mild cold."
C. "This medication helps your body use insulin more effectively."
D. "You may consume alcohol in moderation without worrying."

Correct Answer: C. "This medication helps your body use insulin more effectively."

Rationale:

- **Metformin** improves insulin sensitivity and decreases hepatic glucose production.
- It is generally taken with meals to reduce GI side effects.
- Alcohol intake should be limited; it can increase the risk of lactic acidosis.
- There's no reason to stop for a mild cold.

Q14.

A client has been prescribed a nitroglycerin patch for angina. Which instruction is **most important**?

A. "Apply the patch to the same site daily for consistent absorption."
B. "Remove the patch at bedtime and reapply a new one in the morning."
C. "You can cut the patch to adjust the dosage."
D. "Stop taking sublingual nitroglycerin since you're using a patch now."

Correct Answer: B. "Remove the patch at bedtime and reapply a new one in the morning."

Rationale:

- **Nitroglycerin patches** are typically worn for about 12–14 hours, then removed to provide a "nitrate-free" interval and reduce tolerance.
- Rotating sites prevents skin irritation.
- The patch should **not be cut** to adjust dosage.
- Sublingual NTG can still be used for acute chest pain.

Q15.

A client taking lithium for bipolar disorder has a lithium level of 2.1 mEq/L. Which symptom is the nurse **most likely** to observe?

A. Excessive salivation
B. Slurred speech and ataxia
C. Constipation
D. Alopecia

Correct Answer: B. Slurred speech and ataxia

Rationale:

- A lithium level of **2.1 mEq/L** is above the therapeutic range (0.6–1.2 mEq/L) and indicates toxicity. Signs include **neurological impairment** such as slurred speech, confusion, ataxia, and possible coarse tremors.
- Excessive salivation and constipation are not typical lithium toxicity symptoms.
- Alopecia is not commonly associated with lithium toxicity.

Q16.

A client with atrial fibrillation is prescribed warfarin. The nurse instructs the client to avoid which over-the-counter (OTC) medication?

A. Acetaminophen (Tylenol)
B. Loperamide (Imodium)
C. Ibuprofen (Advil, Motrin)
D. Guaifenesin (Mucinex)

Correct Answer: C. Ibuprofen (Advil, Motrin)

Rationale:

- **NSAIDs** (ibuprofen) increase bleeding risk when taken with **warfarin**. They also can affect platelet aggregation.
- Acetaminophen is safer, though in very high doses it can also affect INR.
- Loperamide and guaifenesin do not significantly affect anticoagulation.

Q17.

A hospitalized client has a continuous IV infusion of morphine for severe pain. The nurse notes the client's respiratory rate is 8 breaths/min. What is the **immediate** nursing action?

A. Discontinue the IV morphine infusion
B. Slow the rate of infusion and reassess
C. Administer naloxone (Narcan) per protocol
D. Call the provider for new orders

Correct Answer: C. Administer naloxone (Narcan) per protocol

Rationale:

- A respiratory rate of 8 indicates **respiratory depression. Naloxone** is the opioid antagonist used to reverse life-threatening respiratory depression.
- Discontinuing the infusion and calling the provider will happen, but the **immediate** life-saving measure is to reverse the opioid effect.

Q18.

A nurse provides teaching to a client receiving spironolactone. Which statement by the client indicates a need for **further** teaching?

A. "I will avoid high-potassium foods like bananas and spinach."
B. "I should report if I notice palpitations or muscle weakness."
C. "If I miss a dose, I can double up the next dose to catch up."
D. "I will have my potassium levels checked periodically."

Correct Answer: C. "If I miss a dose, I can double up the next dose to catch up."

Rationale:

- Clients taking **potassium-sparing diuretics** (spironolactone) must not double up doses if one is missed. This could cause hyperkalemia or other complications.
- Avoiding high-K^+ foods, reporting palpitations (possible hyperkalemia), and periodic lab checks are correct instructions.

Q19.

An elderly client is on digoxin. Which condition predisposes the client to digoxin toxicity?

A. Hypokalemia
B. Hypernatremia
C. Hyperglycemia
D. Hypocalcemia

Correct Answer: A. Hypokalemia

Rationale:

- **Low potassium** levels enhance the effects of digoxin on myocardial cells, increasing the risk for **digoxin toxicity** (nausea, vision changes, arrhythmias).
- Hypernatremia, hyperglycemia, and hypocalcemia are not the classic electrolyte disturbances associated with digoxin toxicity.

Q20.

A client is prescribed albuterol (a short-acting β2-agonist) via an inhaler. Which common side effect should the nurse discuss with the client?

A. Drowsiness
B. Bradycardia
C. Nervousness and tachycardia
D. Hypoglycemia

Correct Answer: C. Nervousness and tachycardia

Rationale:

- **Albuterol** stimulates β2 receptors but can also affect β1 receptors in the heart, causing **increased heart rate**, tremors, and nervousness.
- Drowsiness and bradycardia are unlikely.
- Hypoglycemia is not a typical side effect of albuterol.

Q21.

A client with Parkinson's disease is prescribed carbidopa-levodopa. Which instruction is **most appropriate**?

A. "Take this medication with a protein-rich meal for best absorption."
B. "You may notice that your urine or sweat becomes darker in color."
C. "Double the dose if you feel an increase in tremors."
D. "Stop the drug immediately if you have dizziness."

Correct Answer: B. "You may notice that your urine or sweat becomes darker in color."

Rationale:

- **Carbidopa-levodopa** can cause dark discoloration of body fluids.
- High-protein meals can interfere with medication absorption.
- Dosing changes should not be made independently.
- Mild dizziness can occur; stopping the drug abruptly can worsen Parkinsonian symptoms.

Q22.

A client on long-term corticosteroid therapy (prednisone) should be monitored for which adverse effect?

A. Bradycardia
B. Hyperglycemia
C. Hyperkalemia
D. Hypotension

Correct Answer: B. Hyperglycemia

Rationale:

- **Corticosteroids** can cause **elevated blood glucose levels** and other side effects like osteoporosis, mood changes, fluid retention, and risk of infection.
- They do not typically cause bradycardia or hyperkalemia; they can cause hypokalemia.
- Hypertension, not hypotension, is more common.

Q23.

A client with depression is started on an SSRI (sertraline). Which teaching is **most important** to include?

A. "You'll see improvement in your symptoms within 24 hours."
B. "Avoid drinking grapefruit juice while on this medication."
C. "It may take several weeks to feel the full effect of this drug."
D. "Stop the medication if you experience mild headache."

Correct Answer: C. "It may take several weeks to feel the full effect of this drug."

Rationale:

- SSRIs often take **2–4 weeks** or longer for full therapeutic effect.
- Stopping medication for mild side effects is not advised.
- Grapefruit juice mainly affects certain other drugs; while caution is wise, it's not the primary teaching point.
- Improvement in 24 hours is unrealistic for antidepressants.

Q24.

A client has been prescribed a transdermal fentanyl patch. Which statement by the client indicates correct understanding?

A. "I can use a heating pad directly over the patch to help absorption."
B. "I should rotate sites but can reapply to the same site if no redness."
C. "It's okay to cut the patch if I need to adjust the dose."
D. "I will remove the old patch before placing a new one."

Correct Answer: D. "I will remove the old patch before placing a new one."

Rationale:

- **Transdermal patches** should never be cut, and old patches must be removed to avoid overdose.
- Applying heat can dramatically increase fentanyl absorption, risking toxicity.
- Rotating sites is recommended, but always remove the old patch first.

Q25.

A client with migraines is prescribed sumatriptan. Which client history finding would cause the nurse to question the prescription?

A. History of hypertension
B. History of hypothyroidism
C. Occasional tension headaches
D. Chronic bronchitis

Correct Answer: A. History of hypertension

Rationale:

- **Sumatriptan** is contraindicated or used cautiously in clients with **uncontrolled hypertension** or significant cardiovascular disease because it causes vasoconstriction.
- Hypothyroidism, tension headaches, and bronchitis are not direct contraindications.

Q26.

A client is prescribed enoxaparin (low-molecular-weight heparin). Which teaching point is correct?

A. "This medication does not require routine blood monitoring like aPTT."
B. "A massage at the injection site helps absorption."
C. "If I see small bruises around the injection site, I should stop the injections."
D. "I can use the same site on my abdomen every day."

Correct Answer: A. "This medication does not require routine blood monitoring like aPTT."

Rationale:

- **Enoxaparin** typically does not require routine coagulation monitoring (like aPTT) that unfractionated heparin does.
- Clients should not massage the site (risk of hematoma).
- Small bruises may occur but are not usually an indication to stop.
- Injection sites should be **rotated**.

Q27.

A client receiving intravenous vancomycin complains of severe itching and flushing of the neck and face. The nurse suspects "red man syndrome." What is the **priority** nursing action?

A. Stop the infusion and notify the healthcare provider
B. Slow down the infusion rate
C. Administer an antihistamine and continue the infusion
D. Assess for infiltration at the IV site

Correct Answer: B. Slow down the infusion rate

Rationale:

- **Red man syndrome** is often related to rapid infusion of vancomycin. Slowing the rate and administering antihistamines can help.
- It's not necessarily an allergic reaction that requires the infusion to be stopped completely unless symptoms are severe or anaphylaxis is suspected.

Q28.

A client is discharged on levothyroxine for hypothyroidism. Which instruction is essential?

A. "Take this medication with food to reduce stomach irritation."
B. "You may stop taking the medication if symptoms improve."
C. "Take this medication in the morning, on an empty stomach."
D. "Weight gain is expected and normal with this drug."

Correct Answer: C. "Take this medication in the morning, on an empty stomach."

Rationale:

- **Levothyroxine** is best absorbed on an empty stomach, typically 30–60 minutes before breakfast.
- The medication is usually lifelong; stopping it if symptoms improve could lead to relapse.
- Weight gain typically decreases as hypothyroidism is corrected.

Q29.

A client is prescribed amlodipine for hypertension. Which side effect should the nurse educate the client about?

A. Persistent cough
B. Peripheral edema
C. Tachycardia
D. Hypoglycemia

Correct Answer: B. Peripheral edema

Rationale:

- **Amlodipine** (a calcium channel blocker) commonly causes **peripheral edema**, headache, and sometimes reflex tachycardia.
- Persistent cough is more associated with ACE inhibitors.
- Hypoglycemia is not typical.

Q30.

A nurse is administering IV potassium chloride to a client with hypokalemia. Which guideline is **critical** to follow?

A. Infuse the potassium chloride IV push over 5 minutes
B. Ensure the infusion rate does not exceed 10 mEq/hr
C. Mix the potassium in dextrose 5% in water only
D. Administer via IM injection if the IV site is infiltrated

Correct Answer: B. Ensure the infusion rate does not exceed 10 mEq/hr

Rationale:

- **IV potassium** must be given slowly, typically **no faster than 10 mEq/hr** for a peripheral line to prevent cardiac arrhythmias.
- Potassium is never given IV push or IM.
- It can be mixed in normal saline or D5W, but the critical safety measure is the infusion rate.

Q31.

A nurse is assessing a laboring client. The fetal heart rate is 140 bpm with **late decelerations** that began 30 minutes ago. The uterus relaxes completely between contractions, and the client's cervix is 6 cm dilated. What is the **priority** intervention?

A. Increase the IV infusion rate of oxytocin (Pitocin)
B. Place the client in left lateral position and apply oxygen
C. Continue monitoring; these decelerations are expected during active labor
D. Encourage the client to push with each contraction

Correct Answer: B. Place the client in left lateral position and apply oxygen

Rationale:

- **Late decelerations** suggest uteroplacental insufficiency. Immediate actions include maternal repositioning (lateral) and giving oxygen.
- Increasing oxytocin might worsen decelerations.

- Late decelerations are **not normal** and require intervention.

Q32.

A pregnant client in her first trimester complains of nausea and vomiting. Which recommendation is **best** for relief?

A. "Eat three large meals a day to keep your stomach full."
B. "Take your prenatal vitamins on an empty stomach upon awakening."
C. "Try eating dry crackers before getting out of bed in the morning."
D. "Drink large amounts of fluid during meals."

Correct Answer: C. "Try eating dry crackers before getting out of bed in the morning."

Rationale:

- Eating **dry crackers** or bland foods before rising can help alleviate morning sickness.
- Large meals may exacerbate nausea, as can taking prenatal vitamins on an empty stomach or drinking large volumes during meals.

Q33.

The nurse is assessing a postpartum client who delivered 2 hours ago. Her fundus is boggy and displaced to the right. What is the **priority** action?

A. Massage the fundus until firm
B. Encourage breastfeeding immediately
C. Assist the client to the bathroom to void
D. Assess lochia color

Correct Answer: C. Assist the client to the bathroom to void

Rationale:

- A **boggy fundus** displaced to the right often indicates a **full bladder**, which prevents uterine contraction.
- The priority is to have the client **void**, then reassess.
- Massaging the uterus is done if the fundus remains boggy after bladder emptying.

Q34.

A client at 38 weeks' gestation arrives for a nonstress test (NST). The nurse identifies two accelerations of 15 bpm lasting at least 15 seconds over 20 minutes. The baseline fetal heart rate is 140 bpm. How should the nurse interpret these findings?

A. Nonreactive NST
B. Reactive NST
C. Positive CST
D. Negative CST

Correct Answer: B. Reactive NST

Rationale:

- A **reactive NST** requires at least **two accelerations** (≥15 bpm above baseline for ≥15 seconds) within a 20-minute window.
- CST refers to contraction stress test, not relevant here.

Q35.

A client at 32 weeks' gestation reports painless, bright red vaginal bleeding. Which condition should the nurse suspect?

A. Placenta previa
B. Abruptio placentae
C. Vasa previa
D. Uterine rupture

Correct Answer: A. Placenta previa

Rationale:

- **Placenta previa** typically presents with **painless**, bright red bleeding in the second or third trimester.
- **Abruptio placentae** often includes painful bleeding.
- Vasa previa is rarer and can be accompanied by fetal vessel rupture.
- Uterine rupture causes severe pain and fetal distress.

Q36.

A client in labor has an epidural placed. Which finding would **most concern** the nurse?

A. Blood pressure drop from 130/80 to 100/60 mm Hg
B. Inability to feel the urge to push
C. Complaints of itching at the epidural site
D. Feeling warmth in the lower extremities

Correct Answer: A. Blood pressure drop from 130/80 to 100/60 mm Hg

Rationale:

- **Hypotension** is a common and concerning side effect after epidural placement because it can reduce placental perfusion.
- Mild itching can occur and is less concerning.
- A decreased urge to push is expected. Warmth is not typically alarming.

Q37.

A nurse is reviewing postpartum discharge instructions with a client. Which statement indicates **understanding** of teaching related to sexual activity?

A. "I can resume sexual intercourse as soon as my episiotomy stitches dissolve."
B. "I should wait until my lochia has stopped and my healthcare provider says it's okay."
C. "It's safe once I'm home from the hospital, as long as I feel comfortable."
D. "I'll wait at least 6 months before resuming intercourse."

Correct Answer: B. "I should wait until my lochia has stopped and my healthcare provider says it's okay."

Rationale:

- Typically, couples are advised to wait until **lochia has ceased** and the healthcare provider has given the green light. This usually occurs around 4–6 weeks postpartum.
- Option A is incorrect; stitches dissolve at different times, and lochia flow is more indicative of healing.

- **Q38.**

A nurse is explaining newborn care to a parent. Which explanation about preventing heat loss by **conduction** is correct?

A. "Keep your baby away from drafts and vents."
B. "Dry your baby immediately after birth."
C. "Pre-warm the bassinet and avoid placing the baby on cold surfaces."
D. "Place a cap on the baby's head to prevent heat loss."

Correct Answer: C. "Pre-warm the bassinet and avoid placing the baby on cold surfaces."

Rationale:

- **Conduction** refers to heat loss via direct contact with cold surfaces. Pre-warming surfaces prevents conduction heat loss.
- Keeping away from drafts addresses **convection**.
- Drying the baby prevents **evaporation**.
- A cap on the baby's head reduces **radiation** and convection losses.

Q39.

A breastfeeding mother with mastitis is concerned about continuing to breastfeed. What advice should the nurse provide?

A. "Stop breastfeeding immediately and pump only."
B. "Continue breastfeeding or pumping to maintain milk supply and help clear the infection."
C. "Only breastfeed from the unaffected breast."
D. "Apply ice packs before each feeding."

Correct Answer: B. "Continue breastfeeding or pumping to maintain milk supply and help clear the infection."

Rationale:

- **Mastitis** often improves with continued emptying of the breast. It's safe to breastfeed, and it can actually aid in resolving the infection.
- Applying heat (not ice) might help milk let-down.
- Breastfeeding only from the unaffected breast can cause engorgement and worsen mastitis in the affected side.

Q40.

A client who is 28 weeks pregnant with mild preeclampsia asks why she needs to monitor daily fetal kick counts. The nurse explains:

A. "Kick counts help us know if your baby is in distress."
B. "They confirm that your baby's lungs are fully mature."
C. "Kick counts predict if you will need a C-section."
D. "They indicate whether you are going into preterm labor."

Correct Answer: A. "Kick counts help us know if your baby is in distress."

Rationale:

- **Daily fetal movement counts** help assess fetal well-being. A decrease in fetal movement can indicate fetal hypoxia or distress.
- They do not confirm lung maturity or predict need for a C-section or labor onset.

Q41.

A mother of a 4-year-old is concerned because her child has begun to stutter occasionally. Which response by the nurse is **most appropriate**?

A. "This could be a sign of developmental delay. I'll refer you for a full evaluation immediately."
B. "Your child is experiencing normal language development, and this stuttering may resolve on its own."
C. "Let's have the physician prescribe speech therapy as soon as possible to correct this."
D. "That's highly unusual at age 4; he should already speak perfectly."

Correct Answer: B. "Your child is experiencing normal language development, and this stuttering may resolve on its own."

Rationale:

- Occasional stuttering in preschoolers (3–5 years) can be **normal** and may resolve without intervention.
- Immediate referral isn't always necessary unless stuttering is severe,

persistent, or the child becomes extremely frustrated.

Q42.

A parent of a 6-month-old asks when to start introducing solid foods. What is the most appropriate recommendation?

A. "Wait until 1 year of age to introduce any solids."
B. "You can start introducing single-grain cereals around 4–6 months."
C. "Introduce peanut butter first to build tolerance."
D. "Offer a variety of mixed foods right away."

Correct Answer: B. "You can start introducing single-grain cereals around 4–6 months."

Rationale:

- **Solid foods** (such as iron-fortified single-grain cereals) are typically introduced around **4–6 months**.
- Peanut butter is introduced later (around 6+ months) to reduce allergy risk, but not usually first.
- Waiting until 1 year is too late; offering a variety at once is not recommended.

Q43.

A 2-year-old is hospitalized. Which intervention helps address the toddler's developmental needs?

A. Encourage the parents not to visit frequently to reduce dependency
B. Perform all nursing care quickly without explaining
C. Provide a consistent routine or schedule whenever possible
D. Place the child in a room with older children for socialization

Correct Answer: C. Provide a consistent routine or schedule whenever possible

Rationale:

- Toddlers thrive on **routine and consistency**. This reduces anxiety and promotes security.
- Parents' presence is important.
- Explanations, though simplified, are beneficial.
- Placing a 2-year-old with much older children might not meet developmental needs.

Q44.

A 7-year-old is admitted with suspected appendicitis. Which symptom is **most indicative** of a possible perforated appendix?

A. Sudden relief of pain followed by an increase in diffuse abdominal pain
B. Abdominal pain localized at McBurney's point only
C. Low-grade fever with vomiting
D. Rebound tenderness in the left upper quadrant

Correct Answer: A. Sudden relief of pain followed by an increase in diffuse abdominal pain

Rationale:

- **Perforation** of the appendix can cause a sudden temporary relief of pain as pressure is released, followed by a surge in generalized pain due to peritonitis.
- McBurney's point tenderness is typical for appendicitis, but a sudden relief plus diffuse pain strongly indicates rupture.

Q45.

A 10-year-old client with type 1 diabetes mellitus is learning to self-inject insulin. Which statement by the child shows **understanding**?

A. "I'll rotate injection sites within the same area for a week before switching."
B. "I should inject in my muscle before a sports game."
C. "I can reuse the same needle until it feels dull."
D. "I should keep my insulin pens at room temperature for up to 28 days."

Correct Answer: D. "I should keep my insulin pens at room temperature for up to 28 days."

Rationale:

- Insulin pens can generally be stored at **room temperature** up to about 28 days.
- Site rotation is critical; reusing needles is not recommended.
- Injections are typically subcutaneous, not IM.

Q46.

A teenager on chemotherapy has a low absolute neutrophil count (ANC). Which instruction should the nurse reinforce?

A. "Avoid fresh fruits and vegetables; eat only cooked foods."
B. "Stop brushing your teeth to avoid gum bleeding."
C. "You can play contact sports if you wear protective gear."
D. "You can receive your routine live vaccines if they're due."

Correct Answer: A. "Avoid fresh fruits and vegetables; eat only cooked foods."

Rationale:

- **Neutropenic** clients should avoid sources of bacteria or fungi, including fresh produce. Cooked foods reduce infection risk.
- Good oral hygiene is still important, but gently performed.
- Live vaccines are typically contraindicated with severely immunocompromised states.
- Contact sports increase injury risk.

Q47.

A child with croup (laryngotracheobronchitis) presents with a barking cough and mild stridor. The nurse should anticipate which **initial** treatment?

A. Systemic antibiotics
B. High-flow oxygen by mask
C. Nebulized epinephrine and corticosteroids
D. Immediate intubation

Correct Answer: C. Nebulized epinephrine and corticosteroids

Rationale:

- **Croup** is often managed with **nebulized epinephrine** (for airway swelling) and **corticosteroids**.
- Antibiotics are not indicated unless bacterial infection is suspected.
- High-flow oxygen alone won't address airway inflammation.
- Intubation is reserved for severe distress.

Q48.

A nurse assesses a 4-year-old with dehydration. Which finding is **most** concerning?

A. Capillary refill of 3 seconds
B. Output of 1 mL/kg/hr
C. Heart rate of 150 bpm
D. Mildly sunken anterior fontanel

Correct Answer: C. Heart rate of 150 bpm

Rationale:

- A **heart rate of 150 bpm** in a 4-year-old is quite high, indicating significant tachycardia potentially due to dehydration.
- Cap refill of 3 seconds is borderline but not as alarming.
- 1 mL/kg/hr is adequate urine output.
- Anterior fontanel in a 4-year-old is usually closed; mild sunken fontanel typically refers to younger infants. If they somehow still have a soft spot, mild depression is less concerning than severe tachycardia.

Q49.

A child diagnosed with epiglottitis is drooling and has difficulty breathing. What is the **priority** nursing intervention?

A. Examine the child's throat with a tongue depressor
B. Prepare for emergency intubation or tracheostomy
C. Administer a dose of oral antibiotics
D. Ask the parent to have the child swallow some water

Correct Answer: B. Prepare for emergency intubation or tracheostomy

Rationale:

- **Epiglottitis** can rapidly obstruct the airway. The **priority** is to secure the airway.
- Inspecting the throat with a tongue depressor could trigger complete obstruction.
- Antibiotics will be needed, but airway is first.
- Offering water could worsen choking risk.

Q50.

A nurse assesses pain in a 3-year-old. Which pain assessment tool is **most appropriate**?

A. Numeric rating scale (0–10)
B. Faces pain rating scale
C. Visual analog scale
D. Verbal descriptor scale

Correct Answer: B. Faces pain rating scale

Rationale:

- **Preschoolers** often respond best to the **faces pain scale**, which helps them identify the facial expression that matches their pain.
- Numeric rating scales are more appropriate for older children or adults.

Q51.

A client diagnosed with major depressive disorder tells the nurse, "I feel worthless. I'd be better off dead." What is the **best** response by the nurse?

A. "Don't say that. You have so much to live for."
B. "Why do you feel worthless? Let's talk about it."
C. "You sound very upset. Are you having thoughts of harming yourself?"
D. "I understand how you feel; sometimes I feel that way too."

Correct Answer: C. "You sound very upset. Are you having thoughts of harming yourself?"

Rationale:

- The priority is **therapeutic communication** and **suicide assessment**.
- Dismissing the client's feelings or sharing the nurse's own feelings is not therapeutic.
- Exploration of the root cause is secondary to assessing for self-harm risk.

Q52.

A nurse is providing care for a client with schizophrenia who is experiencing auditory hallucinations. What is the **best** intervention?

A. Encourage the client to ignore the voices and watch TV
B. Acknowledge the experience and ask what the voices are saying
C. Confront the client and insist the voices are not real
D. Administer a PRN anxiolytic immediately

Correct Answer: B. Acknowledge the experience and ask what the voices are saying

Rationale:

- The nurse should **acknowledge** the client's reality (they hear voices) and **assess content** of hallucinations for safety (command hallucinations?).
- Telling the client to ignore them or insisting they aren't real can undermine trust.
- Medication may be needed but first assess content.

Q53.

A client with anxiety disorder is practicing relaxation techniques. Which statement indicates effective use of these strategies?

A. "I get more anxious when I try to meditate, so it's not helpful."
B. "Relaxation exercises only work if I use them once a week."
C. "When I feel anxious, I pause and do deep breathing exercises."
D. "I try to distract myself with loud music whenever I'm stressed."

Correct Answer: C. "When I feel anxious, I pause and do deep breathing exercises."

Rationale:

- **Deep breathing** and other relaxation techniques are most effective when used **consistently**, especially during early signs of anxiety.
- Doing them once a week or only using distraction may not be enough.

Q54.

A client with obsessive-compulsive disorder (OCD) repeatedly washes their hands. Which is the **best** approach?

A. Tell the client handwashing is unnecessary and to stop
B. Allow the ritual initially and gradually limit the time spent
C. Restrict all handwashing to promote behavior extinction
D. Encourage the client to wash their hands more frequently

Correct Answer: B. Allow the ritual initially and gradually limit the time spent

Rationale:

- For **OCD** compulsions, **limiting** but **not abruptly stopping** the behavior helps reduce anxiety over time.
- Abrupt cessation can cause intense anxiety.
- Encouraging more frequent washing or restricting it entirely is not therapeutic.

Q55.

A client in a manic phase of bipolar disorder is pacing and shouting. What is the **initial** intervention?

A. Restrain the client physically
B. Offer a PRN benzodiazepine
C. Encourage the client to join a group activity
D. Use a calm, low voice and set clear limits

Correct Answer: D. Use a calm, low voice and set clear limits

Rationale:

- In **acute mania** with escalating behavior, the nurse should maintain **calm communication** and **clear limits** to de-escalate.
- Medication may be next, but the first approach is a therapeutic intervention.
- Physical restraint is a last resort.

Q56.

A client is admitted with anorexia nervosa. Which assessment finding is **most characteristic**?

A. Body weight at or above normal for age and height
B. Intense fear of gaining weight despite being underweight
C. Stable fluid and electrolyte levels
D. Acceptance of a healthy body image

Correct Answer: B. Intense fear of gaining weight despite being underweight

Rationale:

- **Anorexia nervosa** involves an intense fear of weight gain and a distorted body image despite being significantly underweight.
- Fluid and electrolyte imbalances are common.
- They typically do not accept a healthy body image.

Q57.

A client with post-traumatic stress disorder (PTSD) reports frequent nightmares. Which intervention is a priority?

A. Encourage the client to journal in detail about the trauma daily
B. Suggest sedation medication at night
C. Teach relaxation techniques and consider therapy for nightmares
D. Promote avoidance of any triggers that recall the trauma

Correct Answer: C. Teach relaxation techniques and consider therapy for nightmares

Rationale:

- **PTSD nightmares** may be managed with **relaxation techniques**, imagery rehearsal therapy, or prazosin for nightmare reduction.
- Daily journaling about the trauma could worsen symptoms if not done in a structured therapy context.
- Avoidance of all triggers is not a healthy long-term solution; controlled exposure therapy is more beneficial.

Q58.

A client in the ER states, "I'm going to kill myself," and has a plan. What is the **priority** nursing action?

A. Ask the client why they feel that way
B. Stay with the client and ensure a safe environment
C. Give them a phone to talk to a friend
D. Document the statement and notify a psychiatrist

Correct Answer: B. Stay with the client and ensure a safe environment

Rationale:

- A client with a **plan** and intent to harm themselves needs **immediate, direct supervision** to ensure safety.
- Documentation and notification are necessary but secondary to ensuring the client's safety.

Q59.

A client experiencing alcohol withdrawal has tremors and agitation. The nurse should anticipate administering which class of medication?

A. Benzodiazepines
B. Antipsychotics
C. Beta-blockers
D. Opioid analgesics

Correct Answer: A. Benzodiazepines

Rationale:

- **Benzodiazepines** (e.g., diazepam, chlordiazepoxide) are first-line to manage **alcohol withdrawal** symptoms and prevent complications like seizures.
- Antipsychotics or beta-blockers may be adjunctive but not primary.

Q60.

A client with borderline personality disorder engages in self-harm behavior. Which intervention is **most therapeutic**?

A. Offer immediate socialization therapy
B. Use a consistent approach with limit-setting for behaviors
C. Place the client in seclusion for 24 hours
D. Provide constant praise for any behavior

Correct Answer: B. Use a consistent approach with limit-setting for behaviors

Rationale:

- Clients with **borderline personality disorder** benefit from **clear boundaries** and **consistent** limit-setting.
- Seclusion is not automatically indicated.
- Constant praise might reinforce manipulative behavior.
- Socialization therapy can help, but consistent limit-setting is key.

Q61.

A nurse finds a client on the floor next to the bed. After ensuring client safety, what is the **best** next action?

A. Document "client fell" and complete an incident report
B. Notify the healthcare provider immediately
C. Ask the client why they got out of bed
D. Assist the client back to bed without further intervention

Correct Answer: A. Document "client fell" and complete an incident report

Rationale:

- After ensuring the client is safe, the nurse must **document the event** and complete an **incident report** per facility policy.
- The provider will be notified, but documentation and incident reporting is a priority step.

Q62.

A nurse delegates a bed bath to an unlicensed assistive personnel (UAP). Which statement by the nurse ensures **appropriate** delegation?

A. "Please perform a complete bed bath; I don't have time."
B. "Let me know if you notice any skin breakdown during the bath."
C. "You have to do the bed bath exactly how I do it."
D. "Don't interrupt me unless there is a serious emergency."

Correct Answer: B. "Let me know if you notice any skin breakdown during the bath."

Rationale:

- Appropriate delegation includes **clear communication** of tasks and the expected reporting of abnormalities (e.g., skin breakdown).
- The nurse retains accountability for outcomes.

Q63.

A client requires droplet precautions for influenza. Which protective equipment is **essential** when entering the client's room?

A. N95 respirator
B. Face shield and gloves
C. Surgical mask
D. Gown only

Correct Answer: C. Surgical mask

Rationale:

- **Droplet precautions** (e.g., influenza) require a **surgical mask** within 3 feet of the client.
- An N95 is required for airborne precautions (e.g., tuberculosis).
- Face shields and gowns might be added if splash is possible, but the primary barrier is the mask.

Q64.

A nurse is providing discharge teaching to a client with a new colostomy. Which statement indicates **effective** teaching?

A. "I can expect my stoma to remain pale and dusky."
B. "I should change my ostomy pouch every day."
C. "I will clean around the stoma with mild soap and water."
D. "I can eat any foods I want without affecting my stoma output."

Correct Answer: C. "I will clean around the stoma with mild soap and water."

Rationale:

- **Stoma care** includes gentle cleaning with mild soap and water, ensuring the skin is dry before attaching a new pouch.
- A **dusky stoma** indicates compromised blood flow.
- Pouch changes are usually every 3–7 days or as needed, not daily.
- Certain foods can affect odor and output.

Q65.

A new nurse forgets to administer a medication on time and reports this to the charge nurse. What is the **best** initial action?

A. Document the medication was given on time anyway
B. Contact the provider and complete an incident report
C. Tell the nurse to give the dose now and not mention it
D. Discipline the nurse for negligence

Correct Answer: B. Contact the provider and complete an incident report

Rationale:

- In the event of a **medication error** or omission, the nurse must **inform the provider** (in case additional orders or monitoring is needed) and complete an **incident report** for quality improvement.
- Falsifying documentation or ignoring the error is unethical.

Q66.

An older adult client is at risk for pressure injuries. Which intervention is most effective for prevention?

A. Reposition the client every 2 hours
B. Limit fluid intake to avoid incontinence
C. Use a donut cushion on the chair
D. Massage reddened areas vigorously

Correct Answer: A. Reposition the client every 2 hours

Rationale:

- **Frequent repositioning** is key to preventing pressure ulcers.
- Limiting fluid intake may cause dehydration and worsen skin integrity.
- Donut cushions are not recommended; they can impair circulation.
- Massaging reddened areas can cause more tissue damage.

Q67.

A nurse is preparing to insert a nasogastric (NG) tube. The client begins to cough and gag during insertion. Which is the **best** response?

A. Continue inserting to get past the gag reflex quickly
B. Withdraw the tube completely and try again later
C. Pull back slightly and allow the client to rest before proceeding
D. Encourage the client to hyperextend the neck

Correct Answer: C. Pull back slightly and allow the client to rest before proceeding

Rationale:

- **Coughing and gagging** may indicate the tube is in the oropharynx. Pulling back slightly and letting the client recover helps ensure correct placement.
- Complete removal is not always necessary unless respiratory distress occurs.

Q68.

A nurse accidentally punctures their finger with a used needle. What is the **first** action?

A. Immediately wash the area with soap and water
B. Notify the charge nurse
C. Go to the employee health department
D. Report the incident in writing by the end of the shift

Correct Answer: A. Immediately wash the area with soap and water

Rationale:

- The **first action** after a needlestick is to **wash the site** to reduce infection risk. Then report to the charge nurse and follow facility protocol.

Q69.

When administering a blood transfusion, the nurse must remember which **primary** safety check?

A. Warm the blood product to room temperature by the unit heater
B. Infuse the blood product within 6 hours of receiving it
C. Verify the client's identity and blood type with another licensed staff
D. Flush the line with dextrose solution before blood administration

Correct Answer: C. Verify the client's identity and blood type with another licensed staff

Rationale:

- **Two licensed personnel** must verify the **client's ID and blood product** details before transfusion.
- Blood should be infused within **4 hours** maximum.
- Normal saline (not dextrose) is used for flushing.

Q70.

A nurse observes a colleague not washing hands between client contacts. What is the **best** initial approach?

A. Report the colleague to the state board of nursing
B. Discuss concerns privately and remind them of proper hand hygiene
C. Document the incident in the nurse's personnel file
D. Ignore the issue to avoid conflict

Correct Answer: B. Discuss concerns privately and remind them of proper hand hygiene

Rationale:

- **Peer accountability** includes a direct, respectful approach to address lapses in infection control.
- Reporting to a higher authority might be necessary if the behavior continues, but initial direct communication is recommended.

Q71.

A client is scheduled for surgery and the nurse needs to witness informed consent. Which action is **most** appropriate?

A. The nurse explains the surgery in detail and obtains the signature
B. The nurse verifies that the client understands the procedure and then witnesses the signature
C. The nurse signs the form on behalf of the client if they are alert
D. The nurse obtains phone consent from the client's spouse

Correct Answer: B. The nurse verifies that the client understands the procedure and then witnesses the signature

Rationale:

- The provider explains the risks, benefits, and details of the procedure. The **nurse's role** is to ensure the client **understands** and then witness the signature.
- The nurse does not sign on behalf of the client nor provide the detailed

explanation that is the physician's responsibility.

Q72.

A client with a hearing aid complains it's not working. Which should the nurse check first?

A. Whether the volume is turned up
B. If the ear canal is impacted with cerumen
C. The type of battery used
D. If the client stored it in water

Correct Answer: A. Whether the volume is turned up

Rationale:

- When troubleshooting a **hearing aid**, the simplest check is **battery status and volume** control.
- Earwax and other factors might be secondary checks, but volume is the easiest and first to check.

Q73.

A client receiving tube feedings via PEG tube has a residual of 350 mL. Which action is **most appropriate**?

A. Discard the aspirated contents
B. Reinstill the residual and hold the feeding; notify provider
C. Continue the feeding as ordered
D. Administer an antiemetic prophylactically

Correct Answer: B. Reinstill the residual and hold the feeding; notify provider

Rationale:

- Gastric residual of **>250–300 mL** may indicate delayed gastric emptying. **Reinstill** the residual (unless contraindicated) to prevent fluid/electrolyte imbalance, hold the next feeding, and **consult the provider**.
- Discarding content can cause fluid/nutrient loss.

Q74.

A nurse receives a verbal order over the phone from a physician. What is the **best** nursing action?

A. Write down the order, read it back to the physician, and get confirmation
B. Immediately carry out the order and chart it as a telephone order
C. Ask another nurse to listen on another extension and confirm the order
D. Refuse to take verbal orders and request the physician to come in person

Correct Answer: A. Write down the order, read it back to the physician, and get confirmation

Rationale:

- The **read-back** method is a safety strategy. The nurse writes it down, reads it back, and obtains **confirmation** from the prescriber.
- It's appropriate to chart it as a telephone order after confirmation.

Q75.

An unlicensed assistive personnel (UAP) states, "I don't see why we have to wear gloves for every diaper change. It's a waste." What is the **best** response by the nurse?

A. "You're correct. We only need gloves if the diaper is visibly soiled."
B. "Standard precautions require gloves if there's possible contact with bodily fluids."
C. "You should follow the rules or face disciplinary action."
D. "It's hospital policy, and we must always follow it."

Correct Answer: B. "Standard precautions require gloves if there's possible contact with bodily fluids."

Rationale:

- **Standard precautions** mandate protection against any potential contact with bodily fluids.
- Explaining the rationale is more effective than merely citing policy.

Q76.

A nurse is caring for a client with a Foley catheter. Which intervention **reduces** the risk of catheter-associated urinary tract infections (CAUTI)?

A. Maintaining a closed drainage system
B. Irrigating the catheter every 4 hours
C. Disconnecting the drainage bag once per shift to empty it
D. Replacing the catheter daily

Correct Answer: A. Maintaining a closed drainage system

Rationale:

- **Maintaining a closed system** is crucial to reducing infection risk.
- Frequent irrigation or disconnections increase infection risk.
- Routine daily replacement is unnecessary and also raises infection risk.

Q77.

Which task is **appropriate** for the nurse to delegate to a licensed practical nurse (LPN/LVN)?

A. Initial assessment of a newly admitted client
B. Titrating an IV insulin drip
C. Teaching a client about colostomy care
D. Administering subcutaneous heparin injections

Correct Answer: D. Administering subcutaneous heparin injections

Rationale:

- **LPN/LVN** can administer certain medications (e.g., subcutaneous injections).
- Initial assessments, IV titration, and education on new skills are within the RN scope or require RN oversight.

Q78.

A nurse is reinforcing discharge teaching to a client with a new diagnosis of heart failure. Which instruction takes **priority**?

A. "Weigh yourself every morning at the same time."
B. "Reduce your sodium intake to 4,000 mg/day."
C. "Take your diuretic only when you feel swollen."
D. "Exercise once a month to conserve energy."

Correct Answer: A. "Weigh yourself every morning at the same time."

Rationale:

- **Daily weights** are crucial for detecting fluid retention in **heart failure**.
- Sodium intake is typically restricted to much lower than 4,000 mg/day.
- Diuretics must be taken as prescribed.
- Regular low-impact exercise is recommended, not just once a month.

Q79.

A nurse is caring for four clients. Which client should be assessed **first**?

A. A post-op client complaining of mild incisional pain (3/10)
B. A client scheduled for a chest x-ray in 30 minutes
C. A client with new onset confusion and restlessness
D. A client requesting assistance to the bathroom

Correct Answer: C. A client with new onset confusion and restlessness

Rationale:

- **Change in mental status** (confusion, restlessness) could indicate hypoxia, infection, or other acute problems. This is the highest priority.
- Mild pain, scheduled tests, and toileting needs are less urgent.

Q80.

A client complains of right calf pain and swelling. The nurse notes the right calf is warm to touch and measures larger than the left. What is the **best** intervention?

A. Apply a heating pad to the right calf
B. Elevate the leg and notify the provider
C. Massage the calf gently
D. Encourage active range-of-motion exercises

Correct Answer: B. Elevate the leg and notify the provider

Rationale:

- Suspicion of **deep vein thrombosis (DVT)**: The nurse should avoid massaging (risk of embolus), place the leg in a comfortable elevated position, and call the provider.
- Heating pads could worsen inflammation and are not recommended if DVT is suspected.
- Ambulation or active ROM may dislodge a clot.

Q81.

A nurse educator is discussing postpartum hemorrhage. Which factor places a client at **highest** risk?

A. Multiparity (five or more pregnancies)
B. First vaginal delivery
C. Age less than 25
D. Labor lasting less than 6 hours

Correct Answer: A. Multiparity (five or more pregnancies)

Rationale:

- **Grand multiparity** (≥5 pregnancies) significantly increases risk for uterine atony and postpartum hemorrhage.
- Being young or having a rapid labor are not the highest risk factors compared to multiparity.

Q82.

A client with a new tracheostomy has a large amount of thick secretions. Which intervention is **most important**?

A. Encourage the client to cough effectively
B. Suction the tracheostomy tube as needed
C. Increase the humidity of inspired air
D. Teach the client to use an incentive spirometer

Correct Answer: B. Suction the tracheostomy tube as needed

Rationale:

- **Airway patency** is the priority. With thick secretions, suctioning is critical to prevent obstruction.
- While humidity, coughing, and spirometry can help, the immediate concern is removing existing thick secretions.

Q83.

During change-of-shift report, the outgoing nurse states that a client's IV infiltration has resolved. The incoming nurse notices the site is still cool, pale, and slightly swollen. What action should the incoming nurse take?

A. Continue to use the same IV site
B. Elevate the extremity and slow the infusion
C. Stop the infusion and remove the IV
D. Warm the area and keep the IV at the same rate

Correct Answer: C. Stop the infusion and remove the IV

Rationale:

- **Infiltration** is indicated by coolness, pallor, swelling, and pain. The appropriate action is to stop the infusion, remove the IV, and choose a new site.
- Continuing to use the site can worsen tissue damage.

Q84.

A client with pneumonia is placed on airborne precautions by mistake. They actually require droplet precautions. What is the **priority** nursing action?

A. Notify infection control of the error and correct the precaution
B. Continue airborne precautions to be safe
C. Tell the client they need to leave the mask on at all times
D. Cancel all family visits to reduce risk of exposure

Correct Answer: A. Notify infection control of the error and correct the precaution

Rationale:

- **Correcting a precaution error** is essential. The nurse should follow the proper chain of command and ensure the correct type of isolation is implemented.
- Over-isolating can cause confusion and misuse of resources.

Q85.

A nurse is about to administer scheduled morning insulin to a client with type 1 diabetes. The client's blood glucose is 80 mg/dL and they are nauseous. What is the **best** intervention?

A. Administer insulin as ordered and hold breakfast
B. Withhold insulin and notify the provider
C. Administer half the ordered dose of insulin
D. Give insulin and attempt to have the client eat dry toast

Correct Answer: D. Give insulin and attempt to have the client eat dry toast

Rationale:

- Clients with type 1 diabetes generally still need **basal insulin** to prevent ketoacidosis. If the glucose is slightly low but they are able to eat anything (like dry toast or clear liquids), they should do so.
- Omitting insulin can lead to hyperglycemia and ketoacidosis later.

Q86.

A nurse is assisting a client with right-sided weakness to walk using a cane. How should the nurse instruct the client?

A. Hold the cane on the weak side and move the strong leg first
B. Hold the cane on the strong side and move the cane with the weak leg
C. Hold the cane on the weak side and move the cane with the strong leg
D. It doesn't matter which side the cane is on

Correct Answer: B. Hold the cane on the strong side and move the cane with the weak leg

Rationale:

- **Cane use**: The cane is held on the **strong side**, and it is advanced simultaneously with the weak leg. This provides better support.

Q87.

A nurse is preparing to discontinue a peripheral IV line. Which action should the nurse take first?

A. Withdraw the catheter quickly
B. Don gloves and clamp the IV tubing
C. Lower the client's arm below heart level
D. Apply firm pressure on the site before removing the catheter

Correct Answer: B. Don gloves and clamp the IV tubing

Rationale:

- Before removing a peripheral IV, the nurse should **wear gloves** and **clamp** the IV line to prevent fluid spillage or air entry.
- Then carefully remove the catheter and apply pressure.

Q88.

A client states, "I want to see my chart. It's my information." The nurse's **best** response is:

A. "No, you can't see the chart as it belongs to the hospital."
B. "Yes, but let me get the healthcare provider's permission first."
C. "You have the right to see your medical record. Let me check the facility policy."
D. "Why do you want to see your chart?"

Correct Answer: C. "You have the right to see your medical record. Let me check the facility policy."

Rationale:

- Clients have a **legal right** to access their medical records. The nurse may need to follow facility policy for the proper procedure.
- Denying access is incorrect, and asking "why" can seem confrontational.

Q89.

An older client is newly diagnosed with hypertension. Which teaching strategy is **most** effective?

A. Provide written instructions with large print
B. Give all instructions verbally at once
C. Use medical terminology for clarity
D. Tell the family instead of the client

Correct Answer: A. Provide written instructions with large print

Rationale:

- **Elderly clients** may have visual deficits and memory concerns. Written instructions with large print and clear language reinforce verbal teaching.

Q90.

A client with a history of alcohol use disorder has been prescribed disulfiram. Which statement by the client indicates **understanding** of teaching?

A. "I can have a glass of wine at dinner occasionally."
B. "I should avoid aftershave or mouthwash containing alcohol."
C. "If I stop the medication, I can drink alcohol right away."
D. "This medication will cure my alcoholism."

Correct Answer: B. "I should avoid aftershave or mouthwash containing alcohol."

Rationale:

- **Disulfiram** causes a severe reaction with any form of alcohol, including topical products like aftershave and mouthwash.
- It's not a cure; clients must avoid alcohol for at least 2 weeks after stopping disulfiram.

Q91.

A client with active tuberculosis (TB) is being discharged. Which statement by the client indicates **correct** understanding?

A. "I only need to wear a mask in crowded areas for the first 2 days of treatment."
B. "I need to take my TB medications exactly as prescribed for the entire course."
C. "I can stop my medications when I'm feeling better in a few weeks."
D. "I must be on isolation precautions at home and not leave my room."

Correct Answer: B. "I need to take my TB medications exactly as prescribed for the entire course."

Rationale:

- **TB therapy** typically lasts 6–9 months (or longer). Strict adherence is crucial.
- Stopping early can lead to resistant TB.
- Clients usually don't need complete isolation at home if they follow provider guidelines; wearing a mask in public is important initially.

Q92.

A client with a left mastectomy asks why blood pressure should not be taken on the left arm. The nurse's best explanation:

A. "It hurts more on that side due to nerve damage."
B. "We avoid anything that could increase infection or lymphedema in that arm."
C. "There is no valid reason; it's just standard procedure."
D. "We can take blood pressures there if the pressure is low."

Correct Answer: B. "We avoid anything that could increase infection or lymphedema in that arm."

Rationale:

- **Post-mastectomy** clients are at risk for **lymphedema** on the affected side. Blood pressure measurements, IV injections, or blood draws should be avoided on that arm to minimize risk.

Q93.

When administering medications via a nasogastric tube, which intervention is **most** important?

A. Crush all medications together for efficiency
B. Mix medications with hot water
C. Flush the tube with at least 30 mL of water before and after administration
D. Position the client flat to avoid nausea

Correct Answer: C. Flush the tube with at least 30 mL of water before and after administration

Rationale:

- Flushing the NG tube helps ensure patency and prevents drug interactions in the tube.
- Each medication is administered separately with water flushes in between. The client should be positioned with head of bed elevated.

Q94.

A nurse is preparing to catheterize a male client. Which action helps reduce discomfort?

A. Insert the catheter quickly in one motion
B. Ask the client to bear down and exhale during insertion
C. Inflate the balloon while the catheter tip is still in the urethra
D. Keep the foreskin retracted permanently if uncircumcised

Correct Answer: B. Ask the client to bear down and exhale during insertion

Rationale:

- **Bearing down and exhaling** can relax the urinary sphincter and reduce discomfort.
- Inflating the balloon in the urethra causes pain.
- If uncircumcised, the foreskin should be returned to its natural position after catheter insertion.

Q95.

A nurse is teaching a client with frequent urinary tract infections (UTIs). Which statement suggests **effective** understanding?

A. "I will wipe from back to front after urination."
B. "I should urinate immediately after sexual intercourse."
C. "I'll try to limit fluids so I don't have to go often."
D. "Taking frequent bubble baths will help keep me clean."

Correct Answer: B. "I should urinate immediately after sexual intercourse."

Rationale:

- **Voiding after intercourse** helps flush bacteria.
- Wiping front to back is recommended, not back to front.
- Increasing fluids helps prevent UTIs; bubble baths can irritate the urethra.

Q96.

A client with a cast on the right arm complains of increasing pain and tingling fingers. The nurse notes the fingers are cool and pale. Which is the **best** nursing action?

A. Give pain medication and reassess in an hour
B. Elevate the arm on pillows
C. Assess capillary refill and apply warm compresses
D. Notify the healthcare provider immediately

Correct Answer: D. Notify the healthcare provider immediately

Rationale:

- These symptoms suggest **compartment syndrome**: coolness, pallor, paresthesia, and severe pain. Immediate intervention (possibly cast removal) is needed. Delays can cause permanent damage.

Q97.

A client with Guillain-Barré syndrome is experiencing ascending paralysis. Which assessment finding is **most critical**?

A. Dysphagia (difficulty swallowing)
B. Decreased deep tendon reflexes
C. Urinary incontinence
D. Dyspnea or reduced respiratory effort

Correct Answer: D. Dyspnea or reduced respiratory effort

Rationale:

- **Guillain-Barré syndrome** can progress to the **respiratory muscles**, leading to respiratory failure. Checking breathing effort is critical.
- Dysphagia, decreased reflexes, and incontinence are important but less immediately life-threatening than compromised respiration.

Q98.

A client with suspected meningitis has a lumbar puncture. Which finding of the cerebrospinal fluid (CSF) suggests **bacterial meningitis**?

A. Clear CSF with normal glucose levels
B. Elevated protein and low glucose in CSF
C. Elevated glucose and low protein in CSF
D. Xanthochromic (yellow-tinged) CSF

Correct Answer: B. Elevated protein and low glucose in CSF

Rationale:

- In **bacterial meningitis**, CSF typically shows **high protein** and **low glucose**.
- Viral meningitis often shows normal or slightly decreased glucose.
- Clear fluid with normal glucose/protein suggests no infection.

Q99.

A client has been diagnosed with herpes zoster (shingles). Which precaution is **most** appropriate?

A. Contact precautions
B. Airborne plus contact precautions until lesions are crusted over
C. Droplet precautions
D. Standard precautions only

Correct Answer: B. Airborne plus contact precautions until lesions are crusted over

Rationale:

- **Disseminated shingles** or immunocompromised clients with shingles require **airborne and contact** precautions. Localized shingles in an immunocompetent person might require only contact precautions, but the safest approach is airborne + contact if it's widespread or in certain settings.

Q100.

A nurse is caring for a client with myasthenia gravis who has difficulty swallowing. Which teaching is **best** to prevent aspiration?

A. Tilt the head back when swallowing
B. Schedule meals when muscle strength is highest, often after medication
C. Chew food quickly and drink water immediately
D. Lie flat after meals for at least 30 minutes

Correct Answer: B. Schedule meals when muscle strength is highest, often after medication

Rationale:

- **Myasthenia gravis** often presents with muscle weakness that worsens with activity. Eating when the medication (e.g., pyridostigmine) is most effective reduces aspiration risk.
- Tilting the head back can worsen aspiration risk.
- Lying flat after meals increases aspiration risk.

Q101.

A nurse is evaluating a client's ECG tracing and observes peaked T waves. Which electrolyte imbalance does this finding typically indicate?

A. Hypokalemia
B. Hyperkalemia
C. Hypercalcemia
D. Hypocalcemia

Correct Answer: B. Hyperkalemia

Rationale:

- **Peaked T waves** on ECG are a classic sign of **hyperkalemia** (high serum potassium).
- Hypokalemia often shows flattened T waves or U waves.
- Calcium imbalances tend to affect the QT interval rather than T-wave peaking.

Q102.

A client develops a fever and chills during a blood transfusion. Which action should the nurse take **first**?

A. Stop the transfusion immediately.
B. Administer IV diphenhydramine.
C. Slow the transfusion rate by half.
D. Check the client's temperature again in 15 minutes.

Correct Answer: A. Stop the transfusion immediately.

Rationale:

- The **first action** with any suspected transfusion reaction (fever, chills, back pain) is to **stop the blood transfusion**.
- Then notify the provider and follow the facility's transfusion reaction protocol.

Q103.

An adolescent with cystic fibrosis is admitted for a pulmonary exacerbation. Which intervention is **priority**?

A. Low-flow oxygen via nasal cannula at 2 L/min
B. Chest physiotherapy and postural drainage
C. Restricting fluids to prevent fluid overload
D. Providing a high-fat, low-protein diet

Correct Answer: B. Chest physiotherapy and postural drainage

Rationale:

- **Cystic fibrosis** management includes **chest physiotherapy** to mobilize secretions. This is a critical intervention to improve airway clearance.
- Restricting fluids is not recommended; hydration helps thin secretions.
- Clients with CF need adequate calories, often higher protein and higher fat.

Q104.

A client is admitted with suspected bacterial meningitis. Which **isolation precaution** is most appropriate?

A. Airborne
B. Droplet
C. Contact
D. Protective (reverse)

Correct Answer: B. Droplet

Rationale:

- **Bacterial meningitis** (e.g., Neisseria meningitidis) requires **droplet precautions**.
- Airborne precautions are for TB, measles, varicella.
- Contact is for organisms like MRSA, VRE, C. difficile.
- Protective isolation is for immunocompromised clients.

Q105.

A nurse is teaching a client about self-administration of enoxaparin injections. Which site is the **best** for subcutaneous injection?

A. The middle of the anterior thigh
B. The posterior aspect of the upper arm
C. The periumbilical area (love handles) of the abdomen
D. The subscapular area of the back

Correct Answer: C. The periumbilical area (love handles) of the abdomen

Rationale:

- **Low-molecular-weight heparins** (LMWH) like enoxaparin are best given subcutaneously in the **abdomen**, typically in the "love handle" area (at least 2 inches from the umbilicus).
- This site has reliable absorption and less muscle infiltration.

Q106.

A client with hypothyroidism is prescribed levothyroxine. The nurse should monitor for which **adverse** effect indicating over-replacement?

A. Bradycardia
B. Cold intolerance
C. Palpitations
D. Weight gain

Correct Answer: C. Palpitations

Rationale:

- Signs of **excessive** levothyroxine (hyperthyroidism) include **palpitations**, tachycardia, weight loss, and heat intolerance.
- Bradycardia, weight gain, and cold intolerance are signs of inadequate thyroid hormone replacement (hypothyroidism).

Q107.

A client recovering from a myocardial infarction is prescribed a beta-blocker. Which finding indicates this medication is **effective**?

A. Heart rate decreases from 90 bpm to 72 bpm
B. Blood pressure rises from 110/70 to 140/88
C. Client experiences increased urinary output
D. Respiratory rate increases from 16 to 22 breaths/min

Correct Answer: A. Heart rate decreases from 90 bpm to 72 bpm

Rationale:

- **Beta-blockers** (e.g., metoprolol) reduce heart rate and myocardial workload. A mild decrease in heart rate is a desired effect.
- A rise in blood pressure is not typically desired.
- Increased urinary output is not a direct effect.
- Increased respiratory rate isn't indicative of beta-blocker effectiveness.

Q108.

A nurse is assessing a client post-thyroidectomy and notes numbness and tingling around the mouth. Which electrolyte imbalance is most likely?

A. Hyperkalemia
B. Hypokalemia
C. Hypercalcemia
D. Hypocalcemia

Correct Answer: D. Hypocalcemia

Rationale:

- After thyroid or **parathyroid** surgery, accidental removal or damage to the parathyroid glands can cause **hypocalcemia**, often presenting as perioral numbness, tingling, or Chvostek's/Trousseau's sign.

Q109.

A client with a Foley catheter complains of bladder fullness and discomfort. The nurse notes no drainage in the collection bag for the past hour. What is the **best** action?

A. Flush the catheter with 30 mL of normal saline
B. Check for kinks in the tubing
C. Increase the IV fluid rate
D. Ask the client to bear down

Correct Answer: B. Check for kinks in the tubing

Rationale:

- When catheter output **suddenly stops**, the nurse should first look for **mechanical issues** such as kinks or obstruction before taking more invasive measures.
- Flushing or increasing IV fluids is not the first action if the line is simply kinked.

Q110.

A client with atrial fibrillation is taking dabigatran (a direct thrombin inhibitor). Which statement indicates **correct** understanding?

A. "I don't need any routine blood tests with this medication."
B. "I should have my PT/INR checked monthly."
C. "I can skip doses if my heart rate is normal."
D. "This medication is safe in pregnancy."

Correct Answer: A. "I don't need any routine blood tests with this medication."

Rationale:

- **Dabigatran** and other direct oral anticoagulants do not require frequent INR checks like warfarin does.
- It is not typically recommended in pregnancy.
- Skipping doses is unsafe due to stroke risk in atrial fibrillation.

Q111.

A nurse is teaching a postpartum mother about newborn care. She asks how to clean the umbilical cord stump. The most appropriate teaching is:

A. "Use alcohol swabs around the cord after every diaper change."
B. "Use warm water only; avoid alcohol or antiseptics."
C. "Apply antibiotic ointment on the stump daily."
D. "Clean the area with mild soap and water if soiled; keep it dry."

Correct Answer: D. "Clean the area with mild soap and water if soiled; keep it dry."

Rationale:

- **Current guidelines** often recommend keeping the cord stump **clean and dry**, cleaning with mild soap and water if needed. Alcohol swabbing is not always necessary. Antibiotic ointments are generally not routine unless ordered.

Q112.

A community health nurse encounters a client who states they can't afford the tuberculosis (TB) medications. What is the **best** response?

A. "Stop taking them if you can't afford it."
B. "You only need isoniazid for 2 months if you feel better."
C. "Resources are available; we can help you get the medications at low or no cost."
D. "Let's switch you to a single antibiotic instead of multiple."

Correct Answer: C. "Resources are available; we can help you get the medications at low or no cost."

Rationale:

- **TB treatment** adherence is critical to prevent resistant strains. Public health programs often provide low-cost or free TB meds. Discontinuing or altering therapy is unsafe.

Q113.

A 10-year-old child with type 1 diabetes arrives at the clinic with polyuria, polydipsia, and a blood glucose of 320 mg/dL. The child complains of abdominal pain. The nurse suspects diabetic ketoacidosis (DKA). Which additional finding supports this diagnosis?

A. Bradycardia
B. Fruity odor to the breath
C. Dependent edema
D. Constipation

Correct Answer: B. Fruity odor to the breath

Rationale:

- **DKA** often presents with **ketosis**, leading to a fruity (acetone) breath odor. Tachycardia (not bradycardia) is also common due to dehydration. Constipation and edema are not typical of DKA.

Q114.

A client with stroke who has right-sided weakness is learning to walk with a walker. Which is the **best** teaching point?

A. "Move the walker forward, then step with your strong leg first."
B. "Move the walker and the weak leg forward together, then the strong leg."
C. "Put all your weight on your arms before taking a step."
D. "You can use a walker only if you have full arm strength."

Correct Answer: B. "Move the walker and the weak leg forward together, then the strong leg."

Rationale:

- Correct walker use involves **moving the walker and the affected (weak) leg forward together**, then following with the stronger leg to maintain stability.

Q115.

A child is brought to the ER with suspected acute epiglottitis. The nurse notes drooling, high fever, and the child is sitting upright leaning forward. What is the **priority**?

A. Give oral fluids to prevent dehydration
B. Inspect the throat with a tongue blade
C. Prepare for possible intubation
D. Administer cough suppressants

Correct Answer: C. Prepare for possible intubation

Rationale:

- **Acute epiglottitis** can rapidly lead to airway obstruction. The priority is to maintain a patent airway, often requiring **intubation**.
- Visualizing the throat with a tongue depressor could trigger complete obstruction.

Q116.

A nurse in the mental health unit is caring for a client with bipolar disorder in the manic phase. The client has not slept in 24 hours and refuses to sit still. Which intervention is **most appropriate**?

A. Encourage continuous group therapy to burn off energy
B. Provide a quiet environment and promote short rest periods
C. Give the client a list of tasks to keep them occupied
D. Force the client to stay in bed for at least 8 hours

Correct Answer: B. Provide a quiet environment and promote short rest periods

Rationale:

- In **acute mania**, clients often have **decreased need for sleep**. A quiet environment with short rest periods or naps helps reduce stimulation and encourage brief rest.

Q117.

A client is admitted with a small bowel obstruction. Which clinical manifestation is **most** consistent with this diagnosis?

A. Constant lower right quadrant pain
B. Distention and projectile vomiting
C. High-pitched bowel sounds in all quadrants
D. Painless, bright red rectal bleeding

Correct Answer: B. Distention and projectile vomiting

Rationale:

- **Small bowel obstruction** commonly presents with abdominal **distention** and possible **projectile vomiting** of bile or feculent material.
- LRQ pain is more typical of appendicitis.
- Rectal bleeding suggests lower GI issues.

Q118.

A client with suspected renal calculi (kidney stones) reports flank pain of 9/10. Which provider order is **priority** to implement?

A. Start intravenous fluids at 125 mL/hr
B. Obtain a non-contrast CT scan of the abdomen and pelvis
C. Administer IV morphine for pain control
D. Insert an indwelling urinary catheter

Correct Answer: C. Administer IV morphine for pain control

Rationale:

- **Pain management** is a priority for acute renal calculi. Although imaging and IV fluids are important, addressing severe pain (9/10) is crucial to reduce distress and facilitate cooperation with other interventions.

Q119.

A nurse identifies that a client with dementia is unable to perform ADLs independently. Which intervention **best** promotes autonomy?

A. Complete all tasks for the client to save time
B. Provide step-by-step instructions for each task
C. Encourage the client to do everything independently
D. Restrain the client if they become confused

Correct Answer: B. Provide step-by-step instructions for each task

Rationale:

- Clients with **dementia** often need **simple, step-by-step guidance** to perform ADLs as independently as possible. This promotes dignity and autonomy within their capability.

Q120.

A nursing supervisor witnesses a staff nurse charting medications that were not given. What is the **best** course of action?

A. Warn the nurse privately and forget it
B. Report the incident to the board of nursing
C. Document the observation and follow facility protocol for reporting
D. Confront the nurse and demand an apology

Correct Answer: C. Document the observation and follow facility protocol for reporting

Rationale:

- **Falsifying medical records** is a serious violation. The supervisor should **document** the details and **follow facility policy** for reporting.
- Confrontation alone is inadequate; this is a legal/ethical issue requiring formal action.

Q121.

A 4-year-old child ingests a bottle of chewable vitamins with iron. What is the **priority** nursing intervention?

A. Administer activated charcoal
B. Maintain the child NPO
C. Assess airway patency
D. Contact poison control for guidance

Correct Answer: D. Contact poison control for guidance

Rationale:

- **Iron overdose** can be life-threatening in children. The immediate step is to **contact poison control** or follow emergency protocols, which may include chelation therapy (e.g., deferoxamine).
- Maintaining airway is always essential, but the scenario specifically points to suspected iron poisoning, so immediate poison control guidance is key.

Q122.

A client has left-sided hemiplegia after a stroke and is having difficulty swallowing. What is the **best** nursing action to prevent aspiration?

A. Offer sips of water between each bite
B. Place the client in semi-Fowler's position for meals
C. Tilt the client's head slightly forward while swallowing
D. Provide a straw for all liquids

Correct Answer: C. Tilt the client's head slightly forward while swallowing

Rationale:

- **Head flexion** (chin tuck) helps close the trachea during swallowing and reduces aspiration risk in clients with dysphagia.
- Semi-Fowler's is not enough; high Fowler's is often recommended. Straw use can actually increase aspiration risk in certain dysphagia clients.

Q123.

A nurse is caring for a client with a known latex allergy. Which precaution should be implemented?

A. Use only powdered latex gloves to reduce friction
B. Place a latex allergy alert bracelet on the client
C. Store latex products in a separate compartment in the room
D. Wipe surfaces with alcohol to remove latex residue

Correct Answer: B. Place a latex allergy alert bracelet on the client

Rationale:

- Clients with latex allergy need **clear identification** (bracelet, signage). Non-latex gloves are used. Powdered latex gloves are contraindicated because the powder can spread latex allergens.

Q124.

A client with pneumonia has thick, tenacious secretions. Which measure will help **most** in mobilizing these secretions?

A. Administering IV furosemide
B. Limiting fluid intake to 1 L/day
C. Increasing fluid intake to 2–3 L/day if not contraindicated
D. Keeping the client in supine position as much as possible

Correct Answer: C. Increasing fluid intake to 2–3 L/day if not contraindicated

Rationale:

- **Adequate hydration** helps thin secretions, making them easier to expectorate.
- Furosemide does not directly mobilize mucus.
- Supine position can worsen ventilation.
- Unless contraindicated, higher fluid intake is beneficial for pneumonia.

Q125.

A client who is 8 hours postoperative after hip surgery has a blood pressure of 88/50 mm Hg and pulse 120 bpm. The dressing is dry and intact. What is the **best** nursing action?

A. Administer pain medication and reassess vitals
B. Increase IV fluid rate as ordered and assess for hypovolemia
C. Lower the head of the bed and elevate the legs
D. Check for dependent edema in the lower extremities

Correct Answer: B. Increase IV fluid rate as ordered and assess for hypovolemia

Rationale:

- **Hypotension** and **tachycardia** can indicate **hypovolemia**, especially post-surgery. Even if the dressing is dry, the client may have internal fluid losses or inadequate volume. Increasing IV fluids and assessing volume status is key.

Q126.

A nurse is planning to teach an older adult with hearing impairment. Which strategy is **best**?

A. Shout loudly to ensure they hear
B. Use a lower tone of voice and speak clearly
C. Provide printed materials only
D. Speak quickly to convey information efficiently

Correct Answer: B. Use a lower tone of voice and speak clearly

Rationale:

- Many older adults have presbycusis, with difficulty hearing high-frequency sounds. **A lower pitch** and clear enunciation is most effective. Shouting distorts sounds further.

Q127.

A client with Addison's disease (adrenal insufficiency) is experiencing nausea, vomiting, and confusion. Which laboratory value is most concerning?

A. Sodium 128 mEq/L
B. Potassium 4.2 mEq/L
C. Glucose 110 mg/dL
D. Calcium 9.0 mg/dL

Correct Answer: A. Sodium 128 mEq/L

Rationale:

- Addison's disease can lead to **hyponatremia** and hyperkalemia. A sodium of 128 mEq/L is significantly low and can contribute to confusion.
- Potassium of 4.2 mEq/L is normal, as are the glucose and calcium levels.

Q128.

A mother asks the nurse about discipline for her 2-year-old. Which recommendation aligns with **appropriate** discipline?

A. Reason logically with the child about behavior consequences
B. Time-outs for 1 minute per year of age
C. Physical punishment to teach boundaries
D. Withholding meals if the child misbehaves

Correct Answer: B. Time-outs for 1 minute per year of age

Rationale:

- For **toddlers, time-outs** are an effective, age-appropriate discipline strategy. One minute per year of age is a typical guideline.
- Withholding meals and physical punishment are not recommended.

Q129.

A client has an order for a tobramycin peak level. When is the **best** time to draw a peak level for an IV aminoglycoside?

A. Immediately after the infusion finishes
B. 1 hour before starting the infusion
C. 12 hours after the infusion
D. Right before the next scheduled dose

Correct Answer: A. Immediately after the infusion finishes

Rationale:

- **Peak levels** are typically drawn **30 minutes** (or immediately) after an **IV aminoglycoside** infusion is complete, depending on facility policy, to assess the highest concentration in the blood.

Q130.

A newly licensed nurse is planning care for a client with a chest tube. Which intervention is **incorrect**?

A. Keep the drainage system below chest level
B. Clamp the chest tube when transferring the client to bed
C. Check for continuous water-seal chamber bubbling (if a suction system is used)
D. Encourage the client to perform incentive spirometry

Correct Answer: B. Clamp the chest tube when transferring the client to bed

Rationale:

- **Chest tubes** should generally **not be clamped** unless specifically ordered (risk of tension pneumothorax). It should remain **open** and upright below chest level.
- Checking the water-seal chamber and encouraging spirometry are correct measures.

Q131.

A nurse administers an IM injection to a 2-year-old in the vastus lateralis. Which needle size is **most appropriate**?

A. 18-gauge, 2-inch needle
B. 22-gauge, 1-inch needle
C. 25-gauge, 3/8-inch needle
D. 20-gauge, 2½-inch needle

Correct Answer: B. 22-gauge, 1-inch needle

Rationale:

- **Toddlers** typically need a **22–25 gauge**, 1-inch needle for an **IM vastus lateralis** injection.
- An 18-gauge is too large; 3/8" is too short (subQ needle). 2½-inch needle is usually too long for a toddler's IM injection in the thigh.

Q132.

A client with neutropenia is placed on protective (reverse) isolation. Which intervention is **most** appropriate?

A. Place the client in a negative-pressure room
B. Prohibit fresh fruits or flowers in the room
C. Wear an N95 respirator when entering
D. Group the client with another neutropenic patient

Correct Answer: B. Prohibit fresh fruits or flowers in the room

Rationale:

- **Neutropenic precautions** often include restricting fresh fruits, vegetables, and flowers to limit exposure to bacteria/fungi.
- Negative-pressure rooms and N95 are used for airborne isolation, not neutropenia. Cohorting two neutropenic clients is not standard practice if single rooms are available.

Q133.

A nurse notices that a colleague frequently arrives to work smelling of alcohol. Which action is **most appropriate**?

A. Ask the colleague privately if they have a drinking problem
B. Notify the charge nurse or supervisor about the suspicion
C. Cover for the colleague to keep the unit running smoothly
D. Confront the colleague in front of the team

Correct Answer: B. Notify the charge nurse or supervisor about the suspicion

Rationale:

- Suspected impairment on duty must be reported according to **facility policy**. Safety of clients is the priority. Confrontation in front of peers is unprofessional, and privately asking is insufficient.

Q134.

Which of the following findings indicates effective therapy for a client receiving furosemide for heart failure?

A. Weight gain of 1 kg in 24 hours
B. Bilateral crackles in the lungs
C. Increased urine output and decreased pedal edema
D. Serum potassium of 2.8 mEq/L

Correct Answer: C. Increased urine output and decreased pedal edema

Rationale:

- **Furosemide** reduces fluid overload, so increased urine output and decreased edema suggest efficacy.
- Weight gain and persistent crackles indicate fluid retention.
- A potassium of 2.8 mEq/L is dangerously low.

Q135.

A client with hypertension is prescribed amlodipine. Which side effect is the nurse most likely to emphasize?

A. Dizziness and orthostatic hypotension
B. Frequent urination
C. Persistent dry cough
D. Hypokalemia

Correct Answer: A. Dizziness and orthostatic hypotension

Rationale:

- **Amlodipine** is a calcium channel blocker that can cause **vasodilation**, leading to dizziness and hypotension.
- Persistent cough is associated with ACE inhibitors.
- Hypokalemia isn't typical with amlodipine.

Q136.

A child with leukemia is receiving chemotherapy. Which action should the nurse take to protect the child from infection?

A. Provide fresh fruit and vegetables with each meal
B. Place the child on contact precautions
C. Restrict visitors who have signs of infection
D. Encourage live vaccines to boost immunity

Correct Answer: C. Restrict visitors who have signs of infection

Rationale:

- **Immunocompromised** children must be protected from potential infection sources. Anyone showing infection symptoms should be restricted.
- Fresh produce can harbor microbes; wash or avoid raw produce.
- Live vaccines are contraindicated in severely immunocompromised states.

Q137.

A client reports daily heartburn symptoms unrelieved by antacids. Which recommendation is **best** for managing gastroesophageal reflux disease (GERD)?

A. Eat a large meal before bedtime to prevent nighttime reflux
B. Elevate the head of the bed on blocks
C. Lie down after meals to aid digestion
D. Increase spicy food intake to desensitize the esophagus

Correct Answer: B. Elevate the head of the bed on blocks

Rationale:

- For **GERD, elevating the HOB** helps reduce reflux at night. Avoid large meals before bedtime, and do not lie down immediately after eating.

Q138.

A client at 34 weeks' gestation arrives with painless, bright red vaginal bleeding. Which condition is most likely?

A. Placenta previa
B. Abruptio placentae
C. Uterine rupture
D. Vasa previa

Correct Answer: A. Placenta previa

Rationale:

- **Placenta previa** typically presents with **painless**, bright red bleeding in late pregnancy. Abruptio placentae usually involves painful bleeding and abdominal pain.

Q139.

A school nurse suspects child abuse in a 7-year-old. The child has multiple bruises in different stages of healing. What is the **nurse's legal** responsibility?

A. Notify the parents to discuss the findings
B. Document the bruises and continue observing
C. Report the suspicion to child protective services
D. Ask the child directly if the parents are abusive

Correct Answer: C. Report the suspicion to child protective services

Rationale:

- Nurses are **mandatory reporters**. If child abuse is suspected, the nurse must **contact child protective services**. Proof is not needed; suspicion is enough to report.

Q140.

A client with iron deficiency anemia is prescribed ferrous sulfate. The nurse should teach the client to:

A. Take the supplement with a glass of milk
B. Expect stools to become dark or black
C. Stop taking the supplement if constipation occurs
D. Crush the tablets for better absorption

Correct Answer: B. Expect stools to become dark or black

Rationale:

- **Ferrous sulfate** can cause **black, tarry stools**.
- It should be taken with vitamin C or acidic juice (not milk).
- Constipation is common but can be managed; do not stop abruptly.
- Enteric-coated or extended-release forms should not be crushed.

Q141.

A client with hyperparathyroidism has a serum calcium of 13.2 mg/dL (high). Which symptom is **most** likely?

A. Tetany and muscle spasms
B. Polyuria and flank pain
C. Chvostek's sign
D. Hypoactive deep tendon reflexes

Correct Answer: B. Polyuria and flank pain

Rationale:

- **High calcium** can cause **polyuria** (due to kidney effects) and **flank pain** if kidney stones form.
- Tetany, spasms, and Chvostek's sign indicate low calcium.
- Hypercalcemia can cause decreased DTRs, but kidney-related issues are very common.

Q142.

A teenager with diabetes is learning to administer insulin. The nurse should reinforce:

A. "Inject insulin in the same exact spot daily."
B. "Rotate injection sites within the same anatomical area for a week."
C. "Rubbing the site vigorously after injection improves absorption."
D. "Keep your insulin in the freezer until use."

Correct Answer: B. "Rotate injection sites within the same anatomical area for a week."

Rationale:

- **Site rotation** helps prevent lipodystrophy. Typically, the client rotates among sites (e.g., abdominal quadrants) each week.
- Insulin is not frozen; it should be refrigerated until opened, then room temperature is often allowed for 28 days.

Q143.

A 4-month-old infant is scheduled for an immunization. Which vaccine combination is **appropriate** at this age?

A. DTaP, IPV, Hib, PCV
B. MMR, Varicella, HPV
C. Influenza nasal spray, Tdap
D. Hepatitis A, Hepatitis B, PPSV23

Correct Answer: A. DTaP, IPV, Hib, PCV

Rationale:

- At **4 months**, infants commonly receive **DTaP (diphtheria, tetanus, pertussis)**, **IPV (inactivated polio)**, **Hib (Haemophilus influenzae type b)**, and **PCV (pneumococcal conjugate vaccine)**.
- MMR and Varicella typically start at 12–15 months; HPV is for adolescents.

Q144.

The nurse is caring for a client receiving total parenteral nutrition (TPN). Which intervention is **priority**?

A. Hang new TPN every 48 hours
B. Check capillary blood glucose levels regularly
C. Stop TPN if the bag runs out and start normal saline
D. Administer TPN through a peripheral IV line

Correct Answer: B. Check capillary blood glucose levels regularly

Rationale:

- **TPN** is high in glucose, so **monitoring blood glucose** is essential.
- TPN is typically changed **every 24 hours**, not 48.
- If TPN bag empties prematurely, hang **10% dextrose** to prevent hypoglycemia (not normal saline).
- TPN is usually given via **central line**, not peripheral (due to high osmolarity).

Q145.

A nurse is preparing to administer an intradermal injection for a tuberculin skin test. Which technique is correct?

A. Insert the needle at a 45-degree angle with the bevel down
B. Use a 25-gauge, 1-inch needle
C. Form a bleb (wheal) under the top layer of skin
D. Aspirate before injecting

Correct Answer: C. Form a bleb (wheal) under the top layer of skin

Rationale:

- **Intradermal** injections are given at a 5–15 degree angle with a small 26- or 27-gauge, ¼- to ½-inch needle, forming a **bleb or wheal**. No aspiration is required for intradermal injections.

Q146.

A client with hepatic encephalopathy is prescribed lactulose. Which finding indicates the **drug is effective**?

A. Increased blood urea nitrogen (BUN) level
B. Decreased serum ammonia level
C. Increased mental confusion
D. Elevated bilirubin level

Correct Answer: B. Decreased serum ammonia level

Rationale:

- **Lactulose** lowers **ammonia** levels by promoting excretion in stool, improving mental status in hepatic encephalopathy.
- If confusion is worsening, therapy may be inadequate.

Q147.

A nurse assesses a client with a right arm cast who complains of increasing pain not relieved by medication, and the fingers appear pale. Which complication is the nurse most concerned about?

A. Osteomyelitis
B. Fat embolism
C. Compartment syndrome
D. Reflex sympathetic dystrophy

Correct Answer: C. Compartment syndrome

Rationale:

- **Pain out of proportion**, pallor, and poor perfusion under a cast raise suspicion of **compartment syndrome**.
- This is an orthopedic emergency requiring immediate intervention to prevent permanent damage.

Q148.

A pregnant client states she has been craving laundry starch. The nurse recognizes this as:

A. Normal pregnancy cravings
B. Pica, possibly related to iron deficiency anemia
C. Dysgeusia (altered taste) due to hormones
D. A sign of hyperemesis gravidarum

Correct Answer: B. Pica, possibly related to iron deficiency anemia

Rationale:

- **Pica** is the craving and ingestion of non-food substances (e.g., starch, dirt, ice). It's often associated with **iron deficiency**. Further evaluation is needed.

Q149.

A client with major depression refuses to participate in group therapy. Which approach by the nurse is **best**?

A. "If you don't attend group, you won't get your medications."
B. "It's okay to skip therapy until you're ready."
C. "I understand you're feeling low; can we attend for just 10 minutes?"
D. "Everyone goes, so you have to go too."

Correct Answer: C. "I understand you're feeling low; can we attend for just 10 minutes?"

Rationale:

- A **therapeutic approach** involves acknowledging the client's feelings and gently encouraging participation in small, manageable increments. Forcing or threatening is non-therapeutic.

Q150.

A nurse cares for a client receiving IV heparin for a pulmonary embolism. The client's aPTT is 125 seconds (control 30 seconds). What action should the nurse take?

A. Continue current infusion rate
B. Increase the infusion rate per protocol
C. Decrease or hold the infusion per protocol
D. Add warfarin (Coumadin) to the regimen

Correct Answer: C. Decrease or hold the infusion per protocol

Rationale:

- **Therapeutic aPTT** for IV heparin is typically about **1.5–2 times** the control (~45–70 seconds). A value of 125 seconds is excessively high, risking hemorrhage. The nurse should follow protocol to lower or hold the infusion.

Q151.

A nurse is planning postmortem care for a client who died of suspected Creutzfeldt-Jakob disease (prion disease). Which precaution is necessary?

A. Droplet precautions
B. Contact precautions
C. Standard precautions with additional measures for body fluids and tissues
D. Airborne precautions

Correct Answer: C. Standard precautions with additional measures for body fluids and tissues

Rationale:

- **Prion diseases** require meticulous handling of body fluids and tissues. Standard precautions are typically used, but special care is required for **contaminated instruments** (extended sterilization). Droplet or airborne is not standard for prions.

Q152.

A client is 12 hours postpartum and complains of perineal pain rated 7/10. The nurse notes a firm fundus and moderate lochia rubra. What is the **initial** nursing action?

A. Check for a hematoma on the perineum
B. Administer prescribed oral analgesics
C. Document the findings as normal
D. Call the provider to evaluate for postpartum hemorrhage

Correct Answer: A. Check for a hematoma on the perineum

Rationale:

- Severe perineal pain despite a firm uterus and normal lochia raises suspicion of a **perineal hematoma**. Inspection is necessary first.
- While pain medication may be appropriate, assessing for complications is the priority.

Q153.

A client with a suspected cervical spine injury arrives on a backboard with a cervical collar in place. What is the **best** nursing action?

A. Immediately remove the collar to assess the neck for injuries
B. Maintain immobilization until cervical spine is cleared by imaging
C. Logroll the client every 15 minutes for comfort
D. Obtain a pillow to support the client's neck

Correct Answer: B. Maintain immobilization until cervical spine is cleared by imaging

Rationale:

- **Cervical spine stabilization** must remain in place until x-ray/CT confirms no spinal injury. Early removal can risk permanent injury.

Q154.

A nurse obtains a manual blood pressure of 86/58 mm Hg in an adult client who is stable. Which action is **most** appropriate?

A. Recheck the blood pressure with an automatic cuff
B. Reassess manually in the other arm
C. Immediately call the healthcare provider
D. Begin rapid infusion of normal saline

Correct Answer: B. Reassess manually in the other arm

Rationale:

- If a **low BP** is unexpected but the client is stable, **re-check** with a manual cuff on the other arm to confirm. Then proceed with appropriate interventions.

Q155.

A nurse is changing a sterile dressing on a central venous catheter. Which step is **incorrect**?

A. Don a mask and have the client turn their head away
B. Wear clean gloves to remove the old dressing
C. Clean the site with a circular motion from the center outward
D. Blow on the site to dry it more quickly

Correct Answer: D. Blow on the site to dry it more quickly

Rationale:

- Blowing on a sterile area contaminates it. The site must air-dry or be gently fanned with sterile gauze. Wearing a mask and the client turning away helps reduce contamination.

Q156.

A client states, "I am sure my cancer was caused by evil spirits." The nurse's **best** therapeutic response is:

A. "That's impossible; cancer is caused by genetics or environment."
B. "Tell me more about your beliefs regarding your illness."
C. "Maybe we should get a priest or spiritual leader to exorcise them."
D. "If you believe that, you will have a harder time recovering."

Correct Answer: B. "Tell me more about your beliefs regarding your illness."

Rationale:

- The nurse should use **therapeutic communication** to explore and acknowledge the client's beliefs without judgment. This fosters trust and understanding.

Q157.

A child has pinworms. Which symptom will the parent likely report?

A. Nausea and vomiting
B. Anal itching, especially at night
C. Rash on the trunk and arms
D. Foul-smelling urine

Correct Answer: B. Anal itching, especially at night

Rationale:

- **Pinworms** (Enterobius vermicularis) commonly cause **perianal itching** that is worse at night due to the female worms laying eggs.

Q158.

A client is undergoing an excretory urography (IV pyelogram). Which allergy must the nurse **assess** for?

A. Soy
B. Bee stings
C. Iodine or shellfish
D. Peanuts

Correct Answer: C. Iodine or shellfish

Rationale:

- **IV contrast** used in excretory urography can contain **iodine**, so an allergy to iodine or shellfish is particularly concerning.

Q159.

A nurse is caring for a client with borderline personality disorder who frequently uses splitting behavior. The client says, "You're the only good nurse here; all the others are terrible." The **best** response?

A. "I am flattered you feel that way."
B. "It's not appropriate to say bad things about others."
C. "I understand you feel I'm helpful, but all staff are here to help you."
D. "You're right. Let me speak to the manager about the other nurses."

Correct Answer: C. "I understand you feel I'm helpful, but all staff are here to help you."

Rationale:

- **Splitting** is seeing people as all good or all bad. The nurse should provide a consistent response that maintains boundaries and emphasizes the team approach without reinforcing the splitting.

Q160.

A client's telemetry shows a run of three PVCs (premature ventricular contractions) in a row. They are alert and oriented. What should the nurse do first?

A. Notify the healthcare provider immediately
B. Assess the client's vital signs and oxygenation
C. Prepare for immediate defibrillation
D. Increase IV fluids to flush out the PVCs

Correct Answer: B. Assess the client's vital signs and oxygenation

Rationale:

- First, **assess** the client's status. If the client is stable, gather more data. Runs of PVCs can be dangerous, but immediate defibrillation may not be required unless it progresses to ventricular tachycardia or the client becomes unstable.

Q161.

A nurse is preparing to administer a fleet enema. Which position is **best** for enema administration?

A. Supine with knees extended
B. Prone position
C. Left lateral Sims' position
D. Right lateral Sims' position

Correct Answer: C. Left lateral Sims' position

Rationale:

- The **left lateral Sims'** position helps the enema solution follow the natural curve of the colon. This is the standard for administering enemas.

Q162.

A client with advanced Parkinson's disease has difficulty swallowing pills. The nurse should:

A. Crush pills if allowed and mix with soft food
B. Administer the medication via IV route
C. Skip doses that are difficult to swallow
D. Withhold all oral meds until swallowing improves

Correct Answer: A. Crush pills if allowed and mix with soft food

Rationale:

- Many oral medications can be **crushed** and mixed with applesauce or pudding if they are not extended-release or enteric-coated. This facilitates safe administration in clients with dysphagia.

Q163.

A nurse is providing staff education about cultural sensitivity. Which statement by a staff member indicates **further teaching** is needed?

A. "I should ask clients about any cultural practices regarding food."
B. "I will assume that all members of a certain group share the same beliefs."
C. "It's important to know whether a client uses traditional healers."
D. "Assessing language needs is crucial for good communication."

Correct Answer: B. "I will assume that all members of a certain group share the same beliefs."

Rationale:

- Avoid **stereotyping** or assuming all individuals in a cultural group share identical beliefs. Cultural competence includes individual assessment.

Q164.

A nurse reviews dietary instructions with a client on a low-purine diet for gout. Which food should be avoided?

A. Organ meats like liver
B. Dairy products like milk and cheese
C. Apples and bananas
D. Whole-grain bread

Correct Answer: A. Organ meats like liver

Rationale:

- **Organ meats** (liver, kidney) are high in purines and should be avoided in **gout**. Dairy, fruits, and whole grains are typically acceptable.

Q165.

A client with an ileostomy reports frequent liquid stools. The nurse should explain:

A. "An ileostomy typically drains liquid to semi-liquid stool."
B. "You likely have a stoma infection causing diarrhea."
C. "We can slow it down by decreasing your fluid intake drastically."
D. "You need to flush the stoma daily with normal saline."

Correct Answer: A. "An ileostomy typically drains liquid to semi-liquid stool."

Rationale:

- **Ileostomy output** is naturally more liquid. This is normal; it isn't necessarily diarrhea or infection.

Q166.

A nurse is performing tracheostomy care. Which step is correct?

A. Cut a 4x4 gauze to fit around the stoma
B. Change the tracheostomy ties before cleaning the site
C. Secure new ties before removing the old ones
D. Use cotton-tipped applicators soaked in full-strength hydrogen peroxide

Correct Answer: C. Secure new ties before removing the old ones

Rationale:

- **Prevent accidental decannulation** by securing the new ties first. Do not cut 4x4 gauze (risk of fibers). Typically, sterile trach dressing with a pre-cut slit is used.

Q167.

A nurse is educating a client with peripheral arterial disease (PAD) about foot care. Which statement indicates **need for further teaching**?

A. "I will elevate my legs on pillows to increase circulation."
B. "I should inspect my feet daily for any sores or changes."
C. "I will wear loose, comfortable shoes that fit well."
D. "I'll keep my feet clean and dry, using mild soap and warm water."

Correct Answer: A. "I will elevate my legs on pillows to increase circulation."

Rationale:

- In **PAD**, **elevating legs** too high can actually **decrease arterial perfusion** and worsen pain. Clients often dangle legs to improve blood flow.

Q168.

A nurse is preparing to discharge a client with a prescription for clonidine patches for hypertension. Which instruction is **most important**?

A. "Remove the old patch before applying a new one."
B. "Place the patch below the waistline for best absorption."
C. "You may cut the patch if you need a smaller dose."
D. "Stop using the patch if your blood pressure goes down."

Correct Answer: A. "Remove the old patch before applying a new one."

Rationale:

- **Clonidine patches** must be changed per schedule (usually every 7 days), and the **old patch** should be removed before a new one is applied.
- Avoid placing below the waist; do not cut patches. Do not stop abruptly (risk of rebound HTN).

Q169.

During a mass casualty disaster drill, the nurse must triage multiple victims. Which client is **highest priority** based on the START triage method?

A. A conscious client with a large laceration but normal respirations
B. A client with respiratory rate of 40 and absent radial pulse
C. A client with minor bruises and normal vital signs
D. A client with a closed fracture complaining of pain

Correct Answer: B. A client with respiratory rate of 40 and absent radial pulse

Rationale:

- Under **START triage**:
    - Rapid breathing (>30), absent radial pulse (shock sign), or altered mental status indicate an **immediate** (red-tag) priority.
    - Large laceration but stable vitals might be delayed.

Q170.

A nurse is counseling a client newly diagnosed with HIV. Which statement indicates effective teaching?

A. "I can stop practicing safer sex if my viral load is undetectable."
B. "I should inform sexual partners of my HIV status."
C. "I must donate blood regularly to check my HIV status."
D. "I can share needles with close friends if my viral load is low."

Correct Answer: B. "I should inform sexual partners of my HIV status."

Rationale:

- Clients with HIV **must inform** potential sexual partners, consistently practice safer sex, and avoid sharing needles.
- Having an undetectable viral load does not eliminate transmission risk.

Q171.

A client with acute pancreatitis has severe abdominal pain. The nurse should anticipate which provider order?

A. Clear liquid diet as tolerated
B. Opioid analgesics (e.g., IV hydromorphone) for pain
C. High-fat, high-protein diet
D. Oral NSAIDs only

Correct Answer: B. Opioid analgesics (e.g., IV hydromorphone) for pain

Rationale:

- **Acute pancreatitis** can cause excruciating pain; **opioid analgesics** are indicated.
- Clients are often NPO initially, not on a high-fat diet.

Q172.

A nurse is educating a client on rifampin therapy for tuberculosis. Which statement is **most appropriate**?

A. "If you miss a dose, double the next dose."
B. "Your urine and other body fluids might turn orange."
C. "You can stop taking the medication once symptoms improve."
D. "This medication won't affect your oral contraceptives."

Correct Answer: B. "Your urine and other body fluids might turn orange."

Rationale:

- **Rifampin** can cause orange discoloration of body fluids.
- Doubling a missed dose is incorrect. TB meds require the full course. Rifampin can decrease oral contraceptive efficacy.

Q173.

A client with ulcerative colitis is experiencing 10 to 12 bloody stools per day and abdominal cramping. Which dietary intervention is **best**?

A. High-fiber, raw vegetables to maintain bowel regularity
B. Low-residue diet to decrease bowel stimulation
C. High-fat diet to provide adequate calories
D. Clear liquids only, indefinitely

Correct Answer: B. Low-residue diet to decrease bowel stimulation

Rationale:

- **Ulcerative colitis** flare-ups often require a **low-residue** (low-fiber) diet to reduce bowel irritability. A high-fiber or high-fat diet may worsen symptoms.

Q174.

A nurse prepares to administer timolol eye drops to a client with glaucoma. Which technique is correct?

A. Instill drops directly onto the cornea
B. Instruct the client to blink rapidly after administration
C. Apply gentle pressure to the inner canthus for 1 minute
D. Place the dropper tip on the eyelid to prevent spillage

Correct Answer: C. Apply gentle pressure to the inner canthus for 1 minute

Rationale:

- After instilling eye drops, **gentle pressure** on the nasolacrimal duct (inner canthus) prevents systemic absorption.
- Avoid touching the cornea or eyelids with the dropper to maintain sterility.

Q175.

A client with schizophrenia is standing in the corner, appearing to talk to themselves. The nurse suspects auditory hallucinations. What is the **best** initial response?

A. "What are you hearing right now?"
B. "You need to ignore the voices because they're not real."
C. "I'll give you medicine to stop the voices."
D. "Stop talking to yourself, you're scaring the other clients."

Correct Answer: A. "What are you hearing right now?"

Rationale:

- **Assess** the content of hallucinations first to determine if they are command-type or harmful. This ensures safety and guides interventions.

Q176.

A client with sepsis is receiving IV fluids. Which assessment **best** indicates adequate tissue perfusion?

A. Cool, pale extremities
B. Decreased serum lactate levels
C. Blood pressure of 80/50 mm Hg
D. Urine output of 15 mL/hr

Correct Answer: B. Decreased serum lactate levels

Rationale:

- **Lactate** is a measure of tissue hypoxia. **Decreasing lactate** suggests improving tissue perfusion.
- BP 80/50, low urine output, and cool extremities indicate poor perfusion.

Q177.

A nurse is evaluating client teaching on how to prevent recurrent urinary tract infections. Which statement indicates **correct** understanding?

A. "I will wipe from back to front after using the toilet."
B. "I should void before and after sexual intercourse."
C. "Tight synthetic underwear is best to prevent UTIs."
D. "I should only drink 1 liter of fluid daily."

Correct Answer: B. "I should void before and after sexual intercourse."

Rationale:

- Voiding before and after intercourse helps flush bacteria.
- Wiping front to back is recommended (not back to front).
- Loose cotton underwear is best.
- Adequate hydration is also recommended (usually >2 liters/day).

Q178.

A client with a blood glucose of 35 mg/dL is conscious but shaky and diaphoretic. What is the **best** nursing action?

A. Administer IM glucagon
B. Provide 15 g of fast-acting carbohydrate orally
C. Call the provider
D. Give IV 50% dextrose

Correct Answer: B. Provide 15 g of fast-acting carbohydrate orally

Rationale:

- In **mild hypoglycemia** with the client awake and able to swallow, the **15-15 rule** applies: give 15 g carbohydrate, recheck in 15 min. IM glucagon or IV D50W is for severe or unconscious clients.

Q179.

A nurse is caring for a client with pneumonia who has a new prescription for guaifenesin (expectorant). Which teaching is **most** important?

A. "Decrease your fluid intake."
B. "Take the medication at bedtime only."
C. "This medication will help loosen secretions."
D. "Stop coughing as soon as secretions lessen."

Correct Answer: C. "This medication will help loosen secretions."

Rationale:

- **Guaifenesin** helps **thin and loosen mucus**, promoting airway clearance. Adequate hydration is encouraged. Clients shouldn't stop coughing; productive cough helps clear secretions.

Q180.

A client complains of severe itching after a morphine injection. Which nursing intervention is **best**?

A. Immediately discontinue morphine
B. Administer an antihistamine as prescribed
C. Encourage the client to scratch vigorously
D. Apply a warm compress to the injection site

Correct Answer: B. Administer an antihistamine as prescribed

Rationale:

- **Opioid-induced pruritus** can often be managed with an **antihistamine**. Discontinuing morphine might not be necessary if the itching is not an allergic reaction but a side effect.

Q181.

A client with diabetic neuropathy is at high risk for foot ulcers. Which teaching is **most** appropriate?

A. Walk barefoot around the house to toughen the soles
B. Check feet weekly for cuts or blisters
C. Use a heating pad to keep feet warm
D. Examine feet daily using a mirror if needed

Correct Answer: D. Examine feet daily using a mirror if needed

Rationale:

- **Daily foot inspection** is crucial in diabetic neuropathy. Walking barefoot is risky, and heating pads can cause burns due to decreased sensation.

Q182.

A client with COPD is prescribed pursed-lip breathing exercises. The nurse explains:

A. "Inhale rapidly through your nose and exhale forcefully."
B. "Inhale through your nose for 2 counts, then exhale slowly through pursed lips for 4 counts."
C. "Blow out as hard as you can to empty the lungs."
D. "Use pursed-lip breathing only when you feel short of breath."

Correct Answer: B. "Inhale through your nose for 2 counts, then exhale slowly through pursed lips for 4 counts."

Rationale:

- **Pursed-lip breathing** helps slow exhalation and prevents air trapping. The typical pattern is inhaling for a shorter count and exhaling for a longer count.

Q183.

A 28-year-old pregnant client is concerned about traveling by airplane. She is at 24 weeks gestation. The nurse advises:

A. "Flying is safe during the second trimester; just walk around every 1–2 hours."
B. "You should not fly at all during pregnancy."
C. "You can fly up to 42 weeks if you feel okay."
D. "Flying causes fetal hypoxia, so avoid it."

Correct Answer: A. "Flying is safe during the second trimester; just walk around every 1–2 hours."

Rationale:

- **Air travel** is generally safe during the **second trimester**. To reduce venous stasis, pregnant clients should walk periodically. Most airlines restrict flights after 36 weeks.

Q184.

A nurse suspects a colleague is diverting opioids for personal use. The nurse's **ethical** obligation is to:

A. Confront the colleague privately and warn them
B. Notify the nurse manager or appropriate supervisor
C. Ignore the suspicion unless witnessed directly
D. Ask other co-workers to observe the colleague

Correct Answer: B. Notify the nurse manager or appropriate supervisor

Rationale:

- **Suspected drug diversion** must be reported according to facility policy. It's a client safety issue and an ethical responsibility.

Q185.

A client with Bell's palsy has difficulty closing the eyelid on the affected side. Which intervention is **priority**?

A. Patch the eye 24 hours a day
B. Apply artificial tears and use eye shield at night
C. Massage the eyelid to stimulate nerve function
D. Wear contact lenses to keep the eye moist

Correct Answer: B. Apply artificial tears and use eye shield at night

Rationale:

- **Facial nerve paralysis** (Bell's palsy) can impair blinking, risking corneal drying. **Lubricating drops** and an **eye patch/shield** at night help prevent corneal damage.

Q186.

A nurse is reviewing labs for a client with HIV and notes the CD4+ T-cell count is 198 cells/mm³. The nurse recognizes this indicates:

A. Adequate immune function
B. AIDS-defining criterion
C. Effective antiretroviral therapy
D. Early HIV infection

Correct Answer: B. AIDS-defining criterion

Rationale:

- An **HIV-positive client** with a **CD4+ count <200 cells/mm³** meets the definition for **AIDS** per CDC guidelines.

Q187.

A 50-year-old client is scheduled for a screening colonoscopy. Which instruction should the nurse provide?

A. "You should eat normally up until the procedure."
B. "You'll need to use a bowel prep solution the day before the test."
C. "You can drive yourself home immediately after the procedure."
D. "This test is painful and often requires general anesthesia."

Correct Answer: B. "You'll need to use a bowel prep solution the day before the test."

Rationale:

- **Colonoscopy** typically requires **bowel prep** (e.g., polyethylene glycol) the day prior. Sedation is used, so driving home is not recommended.

Q188.

A client with Addison's disease is started on fludrocortisone. Which finding indicates **over-replacement**?

A. Weight loss and orthostatic hypotension
B. Low sodium and high potassium
C. Hypertension and peripheral edema
D. Hyperpigmentation of the skin

Correct Answer: C. Hypertension and peripheral edema

Rationale:

- **Fludrocortisone** is a mineralocorticoid that can cause sodium and water retention if over-replaced, leading to **hypertension** and **edema**.

Q189.

A newly licensed nurse is caring for a client on contact precautions for MRSA. The nurse asks how to properly remove personal protective equipment (PPE). Which sequence is **correct**?

A. Gloves, gown, goggles, mask
B. Gown, mask, goggles, gloves
C. Gloves, goggles, gown, mask
D. Mask, goggles, gown, gloves

Correct Answer: C. Gloves, goggles, gown, mask

Rationale:

- The **CDC** recommends removing **gloves first**, then **goggles**, followed by **gown**, and **mask** last.
- This prevents contamination of hair/face from heavily soiled gloves/gown.

Q190.

A client has a Jackson-Pratt (JP) drain post-surgery. Which intervention is correct for maintaining the drain?

A. Keep the bulb compressed to maintain suction
B. Empty the drain once daily regardless of output
C. Flush the tubing with 10 mL normal saline every shift
D. Remove the drain once drainage stops for 8 hours

Correct Answer: A. Keep the bulb compressed to maintain suction

Rationale:

- A **JP drain** works by **gentle suction** created when the bulb is compressed. The nurse empties and reactivates suction at least every shift or when half full.

Q191.

A nurse is taking a telephone order from a physician. Which step is **most** important?

A. Immediately carry out the order before reading it back
B. Write the order down, read it back, and get confirmation
C. Ask the physician to text the order to the nurse's personal phone
D. Inform the physician that telephone orders are not accepted

Correct Answer: B. Write the order down, read it back, and get confirmation

Rationale:

- **Read-back** verification ensures accuracy of telephone orders, following patient safety guidelines.

Q192.

A client on a surgical unit is found to have TB. The nurse should:

A. Place the client on droplet precautions
B. Place the client in a negative-pressure room with airborne precautions
C. Use standard precautions only
D. Discharge the client immediately to home isolation

Correct Answer: B. Place the client in a negative-pressure room with airborne precautions

Rationale:

- **Active TB** requires **airborne precautions** in a negative-pressure room. Droplet precautions are inadequate.

Q193.

A post-op client complains of gas pain and abdominal distention. Which action helps promote peristalsis?

A. Encouraging the client to remain supine
B. Providing a straw to drink beverages quickly
C. Assisting the client to ambulate frequently
D. Restricting fluid intake

Correct Answer: C. Assisting the client to ambulate frequently

Rationale:

- **Ambulation** is one of the best methods to stimulate peristalsis and relieve gas pains post-surgery.

Q194.

A nurse witnesses a consent form being signed by a client who received a sedative medication 30 minutes ago. Which action is appropriate?

A. Allow the client to sign; sedation doesn't affect consent
B. Have the client's spouse sign instead
C. Declare the consent invalid and notify the provider
D. Sign as a witness to the client's signature

Correct Answer: C. Declare the consent invalid and notify the provider

Rationale:

- Clients cannot legally give informed consent if they have recently received **sedatives** that could impair judgment. The consent is invalid; the provider must be notified.

Q195.

A client with rheumatoid arthritis is scheduled for physical therapy in the morning but complains of stiffness and pain upon waking. Which nursing action is **most** helpful?

A. Apply warm moist heat to the joints before therapy
B. Encourage immediate vigorous exercise upon waking
C. Provide an ice pack to reduce joint swelling
D. Reschedule therapy for late afternoon

Correct Answer: A. Apply warm moist heat to the joints before therapy

Rationale:

- **Warm moist heat** helps relieve morning stiffness and pain in **rheumatoid arthritis**, improving the client's ability to participate in therapy.

Q196.

A client is receiving doxorubicin chemotherapy. The nurse should monitor for which **adverse** effect?

A. Ototoxicity
B. Nephrotoxicity
C. Cardiotoxicity
D. Hepatotoxicity

Correct Answer: C. Cardiotoxicity

Rationale:

- **Doxorubicin** (an anthracycline) is known for **cardiotoxic** effects (e.g., cardiomyopathy, heart failure). Monitoring cardiac function is critical.

Q197.

A 2-year-old is hospitalized with respiratory syncytial virus (RSV). Which precaution is **most** appropriate?

A. Airborne precautions
B. Contact plus droplet precautions
C. Droplet only
D. Standard precautions only

Correct Answer: B. Contact plus droplet precautions

Rationale:

- **RSV** is primarily spread via **contact** with respiratory secretions, and droplet spread can also occur. Many facilities use **Contact + Droplet** precautions for RSV.

Q198.

An 18-month-old is in the clinic for a well-baby checkup. The toddler's mother is concerned the child can't yet put two words together. The nurse's **best** response?

A. "That's normal for an 18-month-old; many can say several single words."
B. "We need to refer your child for a hearing test immediately."
C. "You should practice flashcards daily."
D. "Children don't usually speak until age 3."

Correct Answer: A. "That's normal for an 18-month-old; many can say several single words."

Rationale:

- By **18 months**, children often have **10+ words** but may not yet combine words. Two-word phrases typically emerge closer to **2 years** (24 months). If severely delayed, hearing tests might be considered, but single-word usage at 18 months is often normal.

Q199.

A nurse observes a UAP placing a restraint vest on a confused client without a physician's order. What is the **best** action?

A. Help the UAP tie the restraint properly
B. Remove the restraint and assess the client
C. Tell the UAP to watch the client closely instead
D. Document the UAP's action in the chart

Correct Answer: B. Remove the restraint and assess the client

Rationale:

- Restraints require a **provider's order** and proper assessment. The nurse should immediately remove an unauthorized restraint, assess the client's condition, and follow facility procedure.

Q200.

A client comes to the ER with slurred speech and right-sided weakness that started 1 hour ago. Which action is **priority**?

A. Prepare for a possible lumbar puncture
B. Obtain a non-contrast CT scan of the head
C. Draw labs for serum potassium levels
D. Administer tissue plasminogen activator (tPA) immediately

Correct Answer: B. Obtain a non-contrast CT scan of the head

Rationale:

- In **suspected stroke**, a **non-contrast CT** is essential to differentiate ischemic from hemorrhagic stroke **before** administering tPA.
- You must confirm no hemorrhage is present prior to tPA therapy.

Final Study Tips

1. **Use the Nursing Process** (Assessment before Intervention unless immediate life-threatening issue).
2. **Prioritize** using **Maslow's Hierarchy** and **ABCs (Airway, Breathing, Circulation)**.
3. **Practice time management** and **focus on rationales**—knowing why an answer is correct (and others are wrong) solidifies your knowledge.
4. **Stay updated** with current guidelines and best practices.

Disclaimer:
These 200 questions are for study and practice purposes only and do not represent official NCLEX items. Always follow your nursing program guidelines and the latest evidence-based practices.

Below are some **commonly used references** for NCLEX-style content and general nursing knowledge. While the sample questions provided in the 200-question set are not drawn verbatim from any single textbook or publication, they reflect the type of content and level of detail found across standard nursing references, guidelines, and NCLEX preparation materials. These sources are widely recognized in nursing education and exam preparation:

1. **NCLEX Test Plans and Official Resources**

   - **National Council of State Boards of Nursing (NCSBN).** (2023). *NCLEX-RN® Test Plan.*
     - https://www.ncsbn.org/exams.htm
     - The official test plan outlines content areas, exam structure, and percentage breakdown for the NCLEX-RN.

2. **Comprehensive NCLEX Review Books**

   1. **Silvestri, L. A.** (Latest Edition). *Saunders Comprehensive Review for the NCLEX-RN® Examination.* St. Louis, MO: Elsevier.
      - A popular comprehensive review guide that includes practice questions, rationales, and test-taking strategies.
   2. **Kaplan Nursing.** (Latest Edition). *NCLEX-RN Prep Plus.* Kaplan Publishing.
      - Provides test-taking strategies, content review, and practice tests with detailed rationales.

3. **Billings, D. M. & Hensel, D.** (Latest Edition). *Lippincott Q&A Review for NCLEX-RN.* Wolters Kluwer/Lippincott Williams & Wilkins.

    - Over a thousand Q&A practice items mirroring NCLEX style, with rationales.

4. **HESI.** (Latest Edition). *HESI Comprehensive Review for the NCLEX-RN® Examination.* Elsevier.

    - Reviews core nursing content with HESI-style questions.

3. Standard Nursing Textbooks

- **Lewis, S. L., Dirksen, S. R., Heitkemper, M. M., & Bucher, L.** (Latest Edition). *Medical-Surgical Nursing: Assessment and Management of Clinical Problems.* St. Louis, MO: Elsevier.

    - Authoritative source for adult health and med-surg nursing topics.

- **Perry, A. G., Potter, P. A., & Ostendorf, W. R.** (Latest Edition).

Clinical Nursing Skills & Techniques. Elsevier.

- o Detailed procedures and clinical skill references.
- **McKinney, E., James, S., Murray, S. S., & Nelson, K.** (Latest Edition). *Maternal-Child Nursing.* Saunders/Elsevier.

  - o Key reference for OB/newborn nursing content.
- **Hockenberry, M. J. & Wilson, D.** (Latest Edition). *Wong's Nursing Care of Infants and Children.* Elsevier.

  - o Pediatric nursing fundamentals and disease-specific care.
- **Varcarolis, E. M.** (Latest Edition). *Foundations of Psychiatric-Mental Health Nursing.* Elsevier.

  - o Covers mental health nursing concepts and therapeutic communication.

4. Clinical Practice Guidelines & Position Statements

- **Centers for Disease Control and Prevention (CDC).**

    - https://www.cdc.gov/
    - Infection control practices, immunization schedules, isolation precautions, and public health guidelines referenced in many NCLEX-style questions.
- **American Heart Association (AHA) Guidelines.**

    - https://www.heart.org/
    - For ACLS, BLS, and emergency cardiovascular care references (used when forming cardiac-related NCLEX questions).
- **American Diabetes Association (ADA).**

    - https://diabetes.org/
    - Guidelines on diabetic management, insulin therapy, and hypoglycemia protocols.
- **Global & National Oncology Guidelines** (e.g., NCCN Guidelines) for cancer care references:

- https://www.nccn.org/

5. Professional Nursing Organizations

- **American Nurses Association (ANA).** *Standards of Practice.*

    - https://www.nursingworld.org/
- **Association of Women's Health, Obstetric and Neonatal Nurses (AWHONN).**

    - https://www.awhonn.org/
- **Academy of Medical-Surgical Nurses (AMSN).**

    - https://amsn.org/

How These References Inform Sample NCLEX-Style Questions

1. **NCLEX Test Plans** from the NCSBN describe the **percentage of questions** on each content area (e.g., adult health, maternal-newborn, pediatrics, mental health, pharmacology). They also detail **client need categories** (safe and effective care environment, health

promotion, psychosocial integrity, physiological integrity) and **cognitive levels** (knowledge, application, analysis).

2. **Comprehensive NCLEX Review Books** and question banks often serve as a blueprint for the **format and depth** of questions. They provide **rationales** that align with evidence-based nursing practice and current guidelines.

3. **Standard Nursing Textbooks** supply the **factual and conceptual knowledge** behind each question's rationale: pathophysiology, clinical manifestations, nursing process (assessment, interventions, evaluation), priority setting, and client teaching.

4. **Clinical Guidelines** from organizations like the CDC, AHA, or ADA reinforce that the information is **current and evidence-based**, particularly for infection control, emergency care, or chronic disease management questions.

5. **Professional Standards** from organizations like the ANA outline

ethical and legal principles, scope of practice, and standards of nursing care, which guide leadership, management, and legal/ethical NCLEX-style questions.

Using References in Your Study

- **Cross-reference** practice questions with the relevant textbook chapter or guideline to confirm the reasoning.
- **Focus** on rationales from trusted NCLEX review books; if a rationale cites a specific guideline (e.g., CDC isolation precautions), look up that **primary source**.
- Keep a **current NCLEX-RN test plan** at hand to understand which categories each question covers.
- Use **multiple resources** (textbooks, guidelines, review manuals) to get a well-rounded understanding of the content.

Disclaimer:

While these references reflect the general sources used in nursing education and NCLEX exam preparation, each practice question set is independently created for review purposes. Always consult your institution's guidelines, course textbooks, and the **latest** official NCLEX test plan for the most accurate and up-to-date information.

www.ingramcontent.com/pod-product-compliance
Lightning Source LLC
Chambersburg PA
CBHW071021240526
45469CB00006BD/2024